Synchronous
NEURAL TIME

by

Marc Kirch

The author claims the right to be credited for ideas formed or sourced in this book.

All rights reserved. This is an original work, not to be amended or emended without the author's written permission or collaboration. No part of this book can be reproduced in any form, or its information stored by any means, electronic or mechanical, without permission in writing from the author.

Copyright Marc Kirch © 2018

ISBN # 9781976811463

Kindle Direct Publishing

Printed in United States of America

Websites referred to in this publication are reviewed and updated periodically, but may not retain the original content or accuracy over time.

"Insofar as we are a mental process, to that same extent we must expect the natural world to show similar characteristics of mentality."

—Gregory Bateson, 1979

Forward

This work presents a somewhat unconventional analysis of current and past experiments that explore the transduction of sensation into perception. Psychophysics, neurophysiology, philosophy, physics, engineering and geometry join here, to show how the spatial organization of neurons and the temporal precision of action potentials give the observer a mental picture of external reality. What is currently a complex, disjointed hodgepodge of experimental facts, which results in part because investigators poke and prod the nervous system with methods that give an oblique view of its function, is assembled and interpreted here into an explanation that is more cohesive. The lack of a controlling paradigm in neuroscience has spawned theories that span the gamut of abstract speculation. However, the theory developed here is directly based on anatomy and physiology and a cogent review of experiments. A book is the preferred method of presentation because ramifications would otherwise be left dangling.

Anyone with an interest in and has a basic knowledge of science should find this narrative understandable. As befits a general audience, the theory is presented with little of the complex analysis that can prevent comprehensive understanding. Jargon is minimized to increase conceptual synthesis and to bridge multidisciplinary boundaries. The reader should not be intimidated by the footnotes as they are required for background but not to understand the ideas as they develop. This account may also be supplemented with internet images and video of, for example, detailed neuroanatomy. Simplified summaries of more important points are at the ends of the first four chapters.

An important sideline of this book is to show how the thoughtful integration of data can create new scientific paradigms. Science isn't all measurements, numbers, and statistical generalizations that create reams of conditional results. Behind the scenes, science should not only seek stimulation with new ideas, but should also reexamine the established concepts that make up its metaphysical foundations. Analyzing data without the imposition of presumptuous traditional explanations can be useful for better scientific principles.

Students are given materials in physics, chemistry and mathematics that due to pedagogical considerations, are presented as problem-solving rules fundamental to understanding. The individuals who originated these scientific laws, such as Pythagoras and Galileo, are thought of as historical gods, though they were curious people who had enough intellectual freedom to toy with intuitive ideas that they were able to develop into formal concepts. The Natural Philosophy of the Middle Ages created scientific rules and concepts that seem primitive now, because the iterative refinements since then have created more specificity and complexity. Scientific order and faithfulness to rules of logic, have created mindsets that are restrictive, because a standard is single by definition. But while many specialized fields are logically consistent internally, we have become accustomed to contrasting methodologies and systems of thinking in overlapping fields of science, such as information theory and neurophysiology, which like adding applies and oranges, create excessive complexity. However, as will be shown, it is possible to find invariants in multiple disciplines, which facilitate integration of nominally dissimilar concepts and facts into a logically consistent theory that has predictive value. Within the theory synthesized here, multiple hypotheses result of varying testability.

This book expands greatly upon a paper written more than three decades ago that explained how the perception of external visual stability arose from convergent neurophysiological mechanisms. While there has been much accumulated research behind the idea that spikes code information, akin to binary-coded packets sent on wires, recent experimental evidence demonstrates that information transfer does not occur for synchronized spikes. The analysis that follows describes the convergence of spikes at synapses, not as a temporal code, but into synchronous timing relationships that match the brain with its sensory environment in graduated stages of spatial convergence. This extended thought experiment, based on large amounts of experimental evidence, may stimulate partisan debates.

The explanations broached in the first chapter are based in part on experiments published more than four decades ago, which described anomalous differences in the cognitive quality of light flicker in visual cortex, compared to the neurophysiological measurements of responses to the same stimulus. This analysis is supported in Chapters Two to Five, in other areas such as somatosensory cortex, hippocampus and the cerebellum. The synchronization of physical, neurophysiological and perceptual time is also discussed in depth. The last chapter examines ancillary but important issues, such as the practice of 'scooping' and how scientific methodology may determine results.

Because this author does not steer established paradigms to account for experimental results, the principles developed here explain without creating systematic complexity. However, rather than over-simplifying with abstractions, detailed arguments are necessary to ultimately show conceptual simplicity, which has practical application as well as elegance. Can the alternative interpretation of neuronal space and time here enable more insight into brain function? Rather than perusing this book by its cover, the curious reader should assess the logic of the novel ideas, then consider whether they warrant the development to the degree presented.

Marc Kirch

CONTENTS

Forward 9

1. How Do Sensory Systems Really Work?. 16

2. Conscious Time and the Sequence of External Events 55

3. Sustained Firing, Continued . . . 70

4. Where Did the Time Go? 130

5. Repetitive Synchrony in the Serial Surfaces of the Cerebellum . . .207

6. Science Friction and the Evolution of Complexity 251

How Do Sensory Systems Really Work?

Currently, it is thought that sensory stimulation by the physical world is converted to moving spikes in neurons, to be reconstituted in our brain as perceptions. Students are taught pioneering concepts like Claude Shannon's Information Theory, Warren McCulloch and Walter Pitts' digital neural logic and the Fourier Transform for encoding and decoding sensory imagery. These basics have resulted in improvements like natural scene analysis, which attempt to meld math and the experience of vision. However, the unquestioned presumptions about neural coding implicit in these techniques have delayed consideration of alternative schemes of the sensation process. Since spiking neurons have evolved independently twice in the earliest multicellular organisms, one expects that this means of communication is not only relatively simple, but since it is conserved in evolution, retains reliability with increased information capacity.[1] Proposed here is a simple and integrative function for spikes traversing organized arrays of neurons, based primarily on evidence in the visual system.[2]

Receptors, whether they be Pacinian corpuscles in the epidermis that sense vibrations, or cones in the retina specifically sensitive to the blue portion of the frequency spectrum of light, transduce an external stimulus into a biological form. They respond selectively to a specific stimulus type in a circumscribed range; the neuron transmits this stimulus sensation centrally with spikes. Increased stimulation intensity results in increased firing rate,[3] resulting in faster temporal summation at convergent synapses, and in turn increasing the speed and intensity of perception in cortex. In the response of retinal photoreceptors to photons, the conformational change induced in rhodopsin molecules is amplified into graded potentials in retinal layers of horizontal cells (in the outer plexiform layer, OPL), then amacrine cells (in the inner plexiform layer, IPL) via bipolar cells that traverse these layers. In the center of the primate retina is the foveola, a region with highest acuity; one cone photoreceptor provides input to

---

[1] Anderson, P., Holman, M., Greenberg, R. (1993) PNAS (USA) 90:7419 show that the phylum Cnidaria (composed of sea anenomes, corals, and jellyfish) has sodium-ion based spikes, very similar to mammalian action potentials. Ctenophora (comb jellies) evolved neurons and synapses independently, but with just glutamate as an excitatory transmitter and fewer neuropeptides; see Hejnol, A. (2014) Nature 510:38.

[2] Occam's Razor states that the simplest solution is the best solution. However, this seems out of date in an era of big data and the perceived hypercomplexity of the brain, now computationally analyzable.

[3] Adrian, E. (1928) The Basis of Sensation; a rate code is an average or median number of spikes in a specified time period; each interval in a train of spikes is a more precise temporal code; a latency code has information in the varied arrival times of spikes at a synapse.

one bipolar Off-cell and one bipolar On-cell, which each contact a midget retinal ganglion cell (RGC) of the same Off or On label on the other side of the plexiform layers.[4] The graded potentials stimulate the emission of spikes, or action potentials (APs), from the RGCs. The RGC afferents bifurcate to the superior colliculus (SC) and the Lateral Geniculate Nucleus (LGN) of the thalamus, major synaptic stations in parallel, which converge in register to the same retinotopic map in visual cortex (V1).

The presumption with any code is that APs transfer information, by virtue of the abrupt amplitude, variable frequency and speed of spikes. However, to funnel the visual detail encoded by ~100 million retinal receptors in humans, into ~1 million optic nerve fibers, is a neat trick because the maximum spike rate is not sufficient to encode the information in the image within the time needed to perceive, which ranges between 100-200 msec.[5] High RGC spike rates at image edges, and subsequent reduction in spike rates, have inspired algorithms that compress video and photo information, based on the idea that the brain must sparsely code imagery.

That the presence or absence of spikes in a single neuron is not a binary code for light is indicated by the separate activation of spikes in On and Off RGCs by the onset and offset of light, respectively.[6] When an invariant hue of constant luminance shines on both the center and surround fields of foveal photo-

---

[4] Calkins, D., Schein, S., Tsukamoto, Y., Sterling, P. (1994) Nature 371:70; Dacey, D. (1993) J. Neurosci. 13:5334.

[5] Curcio, C., Sloan, K., Kalina, R., Hendrickson, A. (1990) J. Comp. Neurol. 292:497; Barlow, H. (1981) Proc. Roy. Soc. Lon. B 212:1.

[6] de Monasterio, F. & Gouras, P. (1975) J. Physiol. 251:167.

receptors, the graded potentials generate RGC APs at the same low average rate in both center and surround.[7] Can temporal variance in a relatively low RGC spike rate transmit subtle variations in luminance or hue? Apparently, the stimulation of oppositely responsive 'Off' and 'On' RGCs is important to transmit changes in contrast at synchronized times at the same receptor location. So does a single RGC really transmit information in a binary code over time or do spikes have an overlooked role?

This question raises the idea that spikes induced by image edges on the retina actually relay a *location* of the image on neuronal axes, rather than constituting a code of image information. Location of a point in space is defined by 3 coordinates, typically x, y and z. On a neural surface, the location of a point in an image can be specified by the x-y position of a cone in the receptor array. Here, spikes are defined as z locations that move with time; sequentially these copy the order of impinging stimulation, rather than confusing that order by summating or averaging over time at synapses. Exaggerated spikes occur whenever a change in contrast occurs, in the image itself or due to fixational eye movements (FEMs), as an image edge crosses retinal receptors.[8] This translation of the z coordinate, while stimulated by edge contrast moving across the cone receptive field (RF), is stated here not to transmit any subtle code over time of graded x-y information in the individual neuron (*Fig. 1*). Spikes in individual neurons here move only location on the

---

[7] Hubel, D. (1995) Eye, Brain, and Vision, pp.40-42.

[8] Microsaccades, drift and tremor, in order of decreasing amplitude, are eye movements that occur during behavioral fixation. FEMs are reviewed in Martinez-Conde, S., Macknik, S., Hubel, D. in Nature Rev. Neuroscii (2004) 5:229.

z axis over distance, without the complication of dimensional properties that change with distance (*Fig. 2*). Stated in simple terms, spikes repetitively move as locations over time down the z axes of neurons, from specific retinal locations where x-y image edge information is defined; image features that become recognized in cortex, are selected by which receptor and RGC types are stimulated. FEMs consisting of microsaccades, drift and tremor, shift the retina across image edges, to stimulate trichromatic receptors and various types of RGCs. Because these selective receptors are a way to spatially organize data, here spikes in an individual neuron are not an organized temporal code of spatial data.

While orthogonal motion in the x-y axes at the retina stimulates the neuronal spikes transmitted down the optic nerve, the actual x-y coordinates of the distant point in physical space where the eyes are

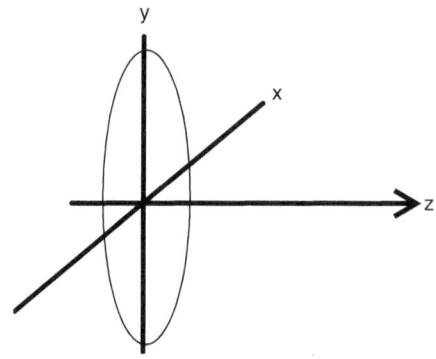

Fig. 1: The x-y axes shown define the retinal surface in one eye. Spikes emitted by RGCs, caused by movements of the retina or stimulus, transmit down the z axis defined by the optic nerve. Complex information in the graded potentials of the plexiform layers is not multiplexed by convergence into an RGC's spike output. Retinal x-y coordinates are defined by an RGC's topographic location relative to the array of RGCs. Because x-y coordinates for any neuron are kept positionally invariant at succeeding retinotopic maps, one spike can transiently move a z location without encoding x-y information.

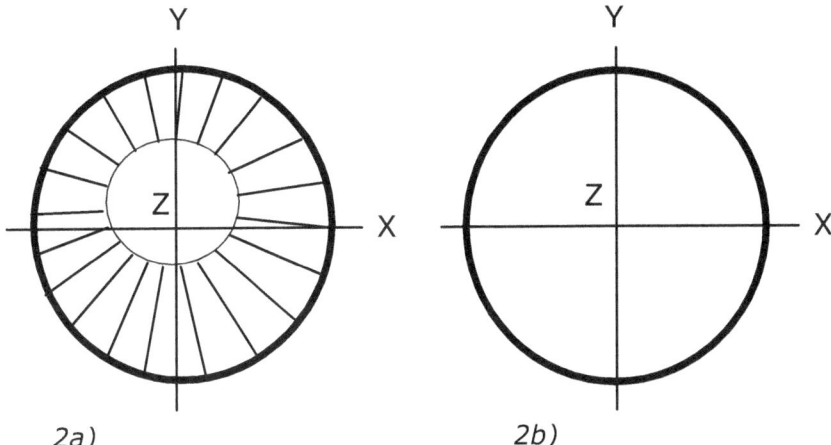

2a)   2b)

Fig. 2a: Translation in the z axis, into the page as you look at this image of a cylinder, creates a diminished circular cross-section with distance. The representation on this page shows two dimensions (2D) projected along the z-axis into three spatial dimensions and time. Fig. 2b: In a 2D world where lines are parallel because dimensions do not contract due to linear or cylindrical perspective, distance cannot be perceived. A circle on the plane of this page, its image reiterated on 2D planes projected on the z-axis, cannot be judged as to distance because the images do not obey laws of dimensional perspective.

fixated, and in the V1 cortical plane, do not move. Foveal cones, during fixational movements, shift orthogonally across the z axis formed by the stable external point where the eyes are fixated and through the image plane in V1, where adjacent neurons converge into large RFs that encompass many shifting foveal RFs.[9] FEMs are actively generated, but the movements of the retina are not countered

---

[9] Motter, B. & Poggio, G. (1990) Exp. Br. Res. 83:37; V1 RF borders do not shift with ocular misalignments of 30 min. of arc. Kjaer, T., Gawne, T., Hertz, J., Richmond, B. (1997) J. Neurophys. 78:3187 find that shifts in fixation point or stimulus position of 10-12 min. of arc within a V1 RF (covering about 1x1 degrees of retinal area in the perifovea) do not change the V1 RF neuronal response. These experiments are consistent with data that show shifting monocular disparities during fixation that are several times larger than the precise fused stereoscopically unshifting image that is perceived, in Westheimer, G. & McKee, S.P. (1978) J. Opt. Soc. Am. 68:450.

to stabilize the image in V1; further discussions in later chapters show that RGC RFs within larger V1 RFs, do not correct subliminal retinal movements via conventional feedback, but via the synchrony of temporally convergent z spikes in perceiving cortex. Still, shifts of the visual field due to head movements are countered by eye movements to stabilize the perceptual location of the peripheral image.[10]

Fixational tremor therefore transiently stimulates specific cone types so that midget RGCs emit spikes proportional to the degree of red, green or blue color intensity (*Fig. 3*).[11] Color-opponent (or Off vs. On) RF center-surrounds converge in V1 and V2 circuits; these afferents integrate a final perception of hue in V4 cortex.[12] The expanded RFs of V4 allow shifting cones in the retinal mosaic to integrate hue from converging neurons and summating APs, without losing the informational resolution at the retina. So what neuronal properties allow the spike to move z location of the image, without also moving its

---

[10] Younge, B., McLaren, J., Brown, W. (2007) J. Neuro-Opthalm. 27:107, prove that with large head tremors, the vestibulo-ocular reflex (VOR) moves the eyes to keep the visual field stable despite the oscillation of the head. Direction-selective RGCs stimulated by both slow and fast head movements, input to the VOR and a cortical accessory optical area to drive eye rotation so that the total visual field is perceptually stable; see Dhande, O. (2013) J. Neurosci. 33:17797.

[11] Inter-subject variability in the ratios of red, green or blue-sensitive cones does not affect the perceptual quality of color; in Hofer, H. Carroll, J., Neitz, M., Williams, D. (2006) J. Neurosci. 26:722.

[12] This color averaging occurs within 10-20 msec (Efron, R. (1973) Perception and Psychophysics 14:518-530), which is near the transit time of a typical microsaccade of 25 msec (Ditchburn, R. (1980) Vis. Res. 20:271). Microsaccades, interspersed with drifts, both span many cone diameters (Martinez-Conde et al, op. cit.). Still, the shifting cone output retains fine spatial and temporal resolution despite order-of-magnitude larger V1 RFs; the convergence of trichromatic retinal inputs occurs in the even larger RFs of V4 cortex, for hue perception (Gur, M. & Snodderly, D. (1997) Vision Res. 37:377).

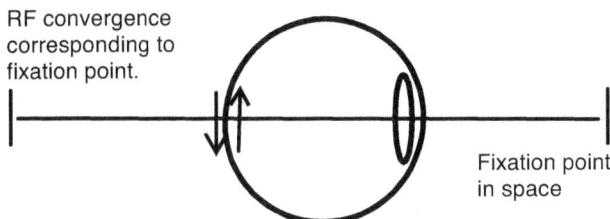

Fig. 3: FEMs cause shifting of foveal cones, shown by arrows in the figure, across the optic, or z axis, while the eye fixates. The cones thus are parallel color filters. Perceived stability during fixation therefore requires an unmoving point in space to stimulate cone RFs and midget RGC APs during FEMs, which converge in much larger V1/V2 cone RFs. Hypothetically, shifting of foveal RGC RFs sustains spikes to convergent synapses in V1/V2 RFs, which create z (but not x-y) stability.

information? The archetypical neuron is designed so that the basic AP is generated in an all-or-nothing fashion that does not change characteristics as it moves down the neuron. The AP that was initiated and now reaches the axon's synapse, is a close approximation in attributes such as speed and shape to a newly initiated spike. In other words, an AP at the proximal end of the neuron has identical properties with other spikes present in the same neuron.[13] By creating a sustained train of spikes,[14] similar repetitive APs, serving as identical markers of location in the z axis, move through first, second and higher

---

[13] AP shape is preserved from dendrites to soma and in a lengthy axon--in Shu, Y., Hasenstaub, A., Duque, A., Yu, Y., McCormick, D. (2006) Nature 441:761. The uniformity of APs has been noted before; see Mukamel, E. & Schnitzer, M. (2005) Neuron 46:357.

[14] A neuron transmits APs at an average speed of 1.8 meter/second between macaque fovea and LGN (Gouras, J. Physiol. 204:407 (1969)). At ~100 spikes/second, 5 spikes may be present in 10 cm length of neuron simultaneously. However, at the LGN one must distinguish between tonic and burst APs: the former are sustained single APs which predominate; the latter are emitted for a short time at a higher frequency but with a long refractory period between the bursts, thus enhancing the ability to fire to new stimuli. These burst APs are induced during inattention and are discussed in Chapter 3. From Sherman, S. (2005) Prog. Brain Res. 149: 107.

order neurons. The z coordinate of the peripheral sensorium is continually in transit as the sustained APs speed to perceptual centers--the map of the retina's sensory surface is exactly in register with corresponding retinotopic maps in cortex in the x and y dimensions, so that the labeled location of an RGC is exactly matched with the corresponding x-y location of an expanded V1 RF.[15] Just as with RGCs, the centers of cortical RFs have an inhibitory surround, which is indicative of competition for horizontal space via lateral processes. This inhibition embodies the dynamic organization of the retinotopic maps in the LGN, SC, V1 and further cortical visual areas.[16] The passage of an AP, or brief pulse of APs, on any z axis is an image marker from an externally fixed x-y location, which, even with convergence in repetitive, larger maps with overlapping RFs, matches the x-y coordinates of the peripheral locus.

Distance cues apparent to the observer are non-existent to the spike. A single neuron does not change the properties of its spikes to confer the property of distance; spike rate or frequency do not change according to where along the length of the axon they are measured. Just as important, stimu-

---

[15] Kara, P. & Reid, R. (2003) J. Neurosci. 23: 8547, demonstrate precise RGC mapping, even with divergence and convergence, to individual neurons in cat V1 cortex. It is necessary that the intermediate LGN stage also is retinotopically precise, shown in Usrey, W., Reppas, J., Reid, R. (1999) J. Neurophysiol. 82:3527.

[16] There are at least 72 topographic maps in macaque cortex, and more in humans; in Perceptual Neuroscience The Cerebral Cortex (1998) by Mountcastle, V., p. 256. At least 16 human visual (retinotopic) maps have been found: in Wandell, B., Dumoulin, S., Brewer, A. (2007) Neuron 56:366. Studies show that the amount of cortical space devoted to peripheral sensations depends on the amount of stimulation that reaches cortex; reviewed in Buonomano, D. & Merzenich, M. (1998) Ann. Rev. Neurosci. 21:149. Cavanaugh, J., Bair, W., Movshon, J. (2002) J. Neurophysiol. 88:2547 examine the spatial dynamics of cortical inhibition.

lation of a single foveal cone cannot determine direction or distance to the stimulus.[17] The cues of linear perspective and motion parallax enable the observer to sense the distance to an object; in one eye, this requires multiple receptors on the retina surface orthogonal to the direction of light into the eye (*Fig. 4*). The greater width between the retinas of the two eyes creates monocular disparities that emphasize stereoscopic three-dimensional (3D) cues for distance and direction.[18] The monocular responses to the same object points generate spikes that converge at specific binocular synapses at the same time; this triangulates distance to the points.

If a receptor or spike cannot discern or code for 'distance', do the laws of physics apply to enable the neuron to intuit distance indirectly? Spatial laws that describe the diminution of measured physical

---

[17] The Styles-Crawford effect is a selectivity for light direction that reduces the response in perifoveal cones to scattered light. An explanation is that collectively, peripheral cones require less sensitivity to scattered light and more selectivity for least-time light for spatial image fidelity. In contrast, cones in the foveola have the least bias for light direction, due to the cone of light focused by the cornea and lens during fixation; see He, J., Marcos, S., Burns, S. (1999) J. Opt. Soc. Am. A 16:2363, and Westheimer, G. (1967) J. Physiol. 192:309.

[18] With 2 retinal points, angle and distance to an object can be triangulated in 2 dimensions, at the same clock time. Motion parallax computes distance by triangulating the position of a moving object on the retinal surface at succeeding times. With 3 retinal points at the same time, one can determine angle, distance and location on horizontal and vertical axes. Other cues for distance, such as shading, haze, occlusion by an object, vergence angle of the eyeballs upon closer objects, and accomodative focus of the lens in the eye, are qualities that require many neurons to perceive. However, when a slender ray of light projects without converging through the narrowed pupil of an eye and its lens, as a parallel beam that impinges onto one locus at the center of the fovea, distance cues are very reduced. Gibson, J. (1979) The Ecological Approach to Visual Perception, discusses 3D perspective and the geometry of distance as 'ecological optics', so that the fastest optical flow is closest to the observer, due to linear perspective and motion parallax that vary with distance.

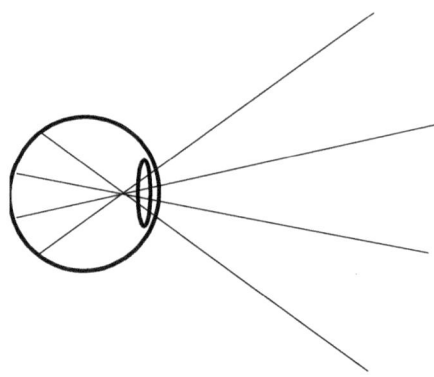

Fig. 4: Linear perspective is shown by the size of an object on the retinal surface that varies with the distance of the object from the eye; the more distant object represented by the 2 inner lines, projects a smaller image onto the retina. The same object, but closer, represented by the 2 outer lines, is converged by the lens into a shorter field of focus and a larger image, thus its distance is more exactly determined. Projected light limited to the z-axis through the center of the lens onto the retina's fovea confers the longest depth of focus and the least amount of visual field converged by the lens.

properties due to the geometry of expansion into space from a point, and the cognitive powers that realize them, are collective properties of many interacting neurons.[19] The solitary foveal receptor has no sense of 'distance' to communicate to its neuron, which fires spikes that are designed to travel to the end of the axon, without a preprogrammed distance or destination. The stereotypical axon of a sensory or motor neuron can be quite lengthy, but with a diameter that is relatively constant. While physical distance laws depend on a central locus bounded by a volume of space, the

---

[19] The law of gravity, Force = Gm_1m_2/r^2, and other inverse-square laws such as Coulomb's law and laws for light luminance, measure a physical property (such as light intensity) in a fixed unit area (such as that measured by a light meter) that declines as the distance squared from a point source into surrounding 3D space. Contrast with linear perspective, as shown in *Fig. 4*, which is a measured change in visual angle that varies inversely with distance.

idealized sensory or motor neuron does not change its cross-sectional area for the length of its axon, as in Fig. 2b. The sense of 3D 'distance' that emerges from our collective neural machinery when we look at a lengthy neuron, is not a fundamental, intrinsic property of axons. The typical axon traverses any objectively measured distance without any change in local 2D geometrical properties. This allows the transfer of the proximal sensation at the receptor, via spikes, which reliably travel to the end of the neuron, so that a spike's 1D quality does not increment with increased axonal length. The orthogonal maps serially traversed by spikes have no intrinsic z-dimension differences between repeated maps connected by topographically aligned neurons.

This basic property of single neurons can be seen on a larger perceptual scale, for example with railroad tracks of constant width that converge optically on the retina with linear perspective. Upon arrival at the distant location of the converging railroad tracks, we find that the width between tracks is identical to that at the location we left. Perspective is created by the convergence of light rays from expansive space onto the small retinal surface, shown in *Fig. 4*, otherwise this surface would need to be the same area as the spatial area perceived, as in *Fig. 2b*. This perspective effect is basic to the Ponzo illusion (spatial expanse that increases due to perspective alters the perception of size, as implied by title lettering on the book cover). A neuron with identical spatial geometry for the length of its axon, also fires identical repeated spikes. Retinotopic maps replicate the x-y position of a neuron's topographic location everywhere on the neuron's z axis, so x-y information is a property of topographical maps not encoded by the z spikes of single neurons.

In fact, the afferent neuron can curve anywhere for any distance without changing the local properties of the peripheral receptor location at the neuron's other end.[20] If a neuron enters into a larger cortical RF from a topographic receptor map, the AP moves z location without changing anything about the receptor location mapped in the larger distal RF.

The repeated maps in the retina, LGN, SC, V1, V2, V3, V4, V5, etc., have precisely mapped topography,[21] a property that is more basic than the three dimensions with which the observer views these repeated surfaces. The surfaces retain approximate area dimensions over distance compared to external space, which converges over many orders of magnitude onto a small retinal surface.[22] That there is a cortical expansion in area, is due to greatly increased numbers of neurons, interneurons and their interconnected synapses, at the same retinal x-y location. An afferent neuron is spatially constrained by equivalent x-y locations along a neuronal z-axis; each neuron is invariantly positioned relative to neighboring neurons, on the sequence of repeated maps. With an ideally invariant cross-section, the neuron's axon without arborizations, has no three-dimensional property (indicated by *Fig. 2b*). This constraint to two dimensions in retinotopically

---

[20] Horton, J., Greenwood, M., Hubel, D. (1979) Nature 282:720, determined that the optic nerve between retinotopic maps is not retinotopically organized.

[21] Besides visual areas, the cortex has repeated auditory, somatosensory and motor maps that preserve the contiguity of peripheral x-y maps; see Kaas, J. & Catania, K. (2002) Bioessays 24:334.

[22] The relative image size of an object, in cortex, is one of several determinants of our perception of distance to an object. See Ungerleider, L., Ganz, L., Pribram, K. (1976) Exp. Br. Res. 27:251. Conversely, Emmert's Law states that perceived distance affects how large we see an area of constant retinal dimensions.

mapped neurons, whose spikes do not code distance differences between retinotopic surfaces, can be referred to as z axis equivalence.[23] This basic precision of retinotopic maps accommodates greater convergence and divergence in larger RFs in distal cortex; adjacent x-y locations that extend processes in orthogonal layers, may integrate related percepts in distally larger RFs over time.

How can sustained spikes support the physical transfer of retinal z location to cortex? Under experimental conditions, with the initiation of a new stimulus, retinal APs last for several 10's of milliseconds. A short stimulus of say, 2 msec, always creates a long period of graded potential activity in the plexiform layers and a long period of maintained discharge from RGCs.[24] Variable stimulus times of 2 through 32 msec duration create the same sustained response duration of about 60 msec in cat foveal RGC's.[25] This indicates that emitted time is shown by one spike or a short burst of emissions from an On-type RGC. If only z-axis loci move as APs move, then the sustained duration does not correspond to stimulus information content, or the time course of the stimulus. The 60 msec of sustained firing may, instead, be necessary to stimulate upper stage neurons to fire by spatial and temporal sum-

---

[23] What is Life (1945), by Erwin Schrodinger, discusses how biological versions of physical law can apply without contradiction; p. 76. Two dimensions make a logical world in Flatland, by E. Abbott (1884).

[24] Levick, W. (1973) Vis. Res. 13:837. Graded potentials in the plexiform layers of the cat retina can last 100 msec at low light intensities, before stimulating the firing of spikes from RGCs.

[25] Levick, W. & Zacks, J. (1970) J. Physiol. 206:677. Cats have a limited frequency of tremor, drift, and microsaccades compared to primates, so that sustained spiking is more likely to be initiated by target movement rather than eye movements; in Martinez-Conde, S. & Macknik, S. (2008) J. Vision 8:28.1.

mation, so that the cortex perceives the peripheral stimulation, even if stimulated duration is short.

Under natural conditions with a constantly shifting retina due to tremor, drift, and microsaccades, one can assume that sustained APs are the norm much of the time in parvocellular (P) neurons from the fovea. Whereas, under experimental conditions that counter these fixational movements by stabilizing the image on the eye,[26] sustained APs result by moving a stimulus edge instead into a receptor's RF. The presumption with electrode recording at stationary locations, is that a spike frequency is a code transmitted from neuron to neuron, in which synapses decode the message that may continue to further stages. However, the z equivalence concept in basic form, states that APs move only emitted z location over time and distance, without coding x-y image information to be decoded at cortical stages. One can elucidate the function of sustained spikes by comparing cones and P RGCs that mediate high resolution vision at the fovea, with the magnocellular (M) labeled receptors and RGCs, which dominate the outer periphery of the retina and fire transiently to edges.[27] A highly detailed image creates a high frequency of edge crossings during fixation, which sustains the emission of many spikes from P RGCs.

In contrast, M RGCs, also known as parasol cells, have large RFs which do not respond to the high resolution of the image. This corresponds with the

---

[26] If the stimulus or all eye movements stop, then sustained spiking will also stop, resulting in lack of vision once visual persistence ends in about 80 msec in humans (Martinez-Conde et al., op. cit.).

[27] Anatomical differences between cat and primate visual systems do not alter the discussion here. See Peters, A., Payne, B., Budd, J. (1994) Cereb. Cort. 4:215 for cortical details; retinal differences are in Wassle, H. & Boycott, B. (1991) Physiol. Rev. 71:447.

initial convergence of many receptors onto single M RGCs. These RGCs are therefore acutely sensitive to movement across the retinal surface and modulate the duration of phasic response according to the amount of stimulus movement.[28] Their precise-duration response from sequentially activated receptors, moves spike locations to cortical area V5 where motion perception occurs; as the motion stimulates each receptor, spikes emit with each incremental input without waiting to summate over the whole RF convergent area. While small foveal RGC RFs in the P system sustain spikes with small fixational edge crossings, in M neurons sustained firing from converging inputs instead indicates the extent of edge movement across the retinal surface covered by a larger RF. The binding of perceived image movement with the detailed object that is moving has to be due to coincident activation of several perceptual maps from the same retinal locus that possess overlapping types of P, M and Off- vs. On-center RGCs.[29] It is also possible that the multiple RGC types converge at the same x-y mapped location but with more synapses in a distal large RF. With fixational pursuit of a moving target, foveal P RGCs respond only to the target and not to the background motion of the field behind the target.[30]

If, as previously asserted, 'distance', either in visual space or in the neuron, is not encoded by one neuron's spikes, then the percepts of 'length' and linear

---

[28] Frechette, E., Sher, A., Grivich, M., Petrusca, D., Litke, A., Chichilnisky, E. (2005) J. Neurophys. 94:119, find that magnocellular RGC spike train times predict stimulus speed across the visual field with an approximate 99% accuracy.

[29] Grunert, U., Greferath, U., Boycott, B., Wassle, H. (1993) Vis. Res. 33:1; Dacey, D. & Petersen, M. (1992) PNAS (USA) 89:9666.

[30] Olveczky, B., Baccus, S., Meister, M. (2003) Nature 423:421.

perspective must issue from light rays on a retinal surface transduced via receptors and APs in neuron arrays.[31] An artifact of neural assemblies dependent on the perception of 3D distance, is the accompanying quality of time. In a 3D world, x-y and the location/time of z coordinates change as a target moves, affecting distance and perspective. Reductionist logic is reversed, because rather than single neurons causing emergent behavior in ensembles of neurons, the ensembles impose global properties.[32] So an observer's 3D neurons perceive a single neuron has 3D properties. However, in the reductionism described here, as a z spike moves, the x and y coordinates stay constant.[33] Perceptual and anatomical 3D results from invariant, repeated 2D maps and the mobile z spike. Fixational tremor stimulates each 2D retinal surface to move z spikes; intuitively, the motion of z spikes past repeated orthogonal x-y surfaces creates an integrated percept from the processional repetition of z locations over time.

RGC spikes that move z location from external image edges, are required to impedance match retinal

---

[31] 'Distance' here, is a perception due to perspective cues and 'length' is an objectively measured distance, and are nominally distinguished when a plane projecting vertically between the cortices of an observer into linear perspective is rotated to be a parallel plane of like length, equidistant from the observer.

[32] Goldman, M., Golowasch, J., Marder, E., Abbott, L. (2001) J. Neurosci. $\underline{21}$:5229. This study shows that the firing properties of individual neurons can be modulated artificially, and also that the global properties of an ensemble will not change, due to compensation by other neurons in the ensemble.

[33] Limiting maps to independent 2 dimensional surfaces that repeat, but do not add into a 3D volume, as stated here, is a dimensional paradigm of neuronal anatomy not to be confused with the minimization of many visual dimensions, or reduction of information, onto the V1 2D cortical surface map, as described in Chklovskii, D. & Koulakov, A. (2004) Ann. Rev. Neurosci. $\underline{27}$:369.

locations with retinotopically mapped cortical locations. A gradual biological matching in vision requires that the retina responds to photonic trajectories of external resolution without image degradation by the aqueous and vitreous humors filling the eye. This matching,[34] defined by the equal resistances of physical transmitting and biological receiving media, is shown by the sensitivity of a rhodopsin molecule in a photoreceptor to a single photon.[35] If graduated matching of successive surfaces were not present, significant numbers of photons would be reflected away at the cornea and lens, reducing the ability of the retina to resolve detail, especially in low-light conditions. Even with light exposure limited by pupil diameter, retinal receptors are responsive to luminance intensities that span several orders of magnitude. Bipolar cells that traverse the plexiform layers have a smaller dynamic response range that saturates faster.[36] At the last retinal stage, plexiform feedback governs output RGCs to a maximum rate of a few hundred spikes/sec.[37] This impedance matched rate responds abruptly to the

---

[34] Mechanical and electrical impedance matching are required in the design of electrodes at neural interfaces, see Micera, S. & Navarro, X. (2007) Int. Rev. Neurobiol. $\underline{86}$:23; neurons and their assemblies also interface in stages that require matching. Biological impedance matching is a gradual change in mechanical or electrical resistance from one medium (or here, neural assembly) to another, so that a stimulus such as photon power, has transmission maximized and reflection minimized; see French, M. (1994) Invention and Evolution, 2nd ed., Chapter Six.

[35] Laughlin, S. (1981) Handbook of Sensory Physiology, $\underline{7}$:6B; Capovilla, M., Hare, W., Owen, W. (1987) J. Physiol. $\underline{391}$:125.

[36] Wu, S. (2010) Inv. Opthalm. Vis. Sci. $\underline{51}$:1263.

[37] Kuffler, S. (1953) J.Neurophys. $\underline{16}$:37; Barlow, (1981) op. cit.; Barlow, H. & Levick W. (1969) J. Physiol. $\underline{202}$:699; light or dark-adapted RGCs respond to a uniformly lit field with a maintained, low spike rate that ramps up an order of magnitude in response to luminance levels that span several orders of magnitude.

high contrast of stimulus edges at a retinal x-y location, to relay z location centrally, rather than sparsely coding subtle edge information that reconstructs the image.[38] Spike shape or timing would have to code image quality perfectly, and otherwise error-correct the retinal image for it to be accurately reconstructed.[39] The equivalence of specific x-y locations on serial retinotopic maps, avoids image degradation due to reduced spike rates and noise, because here, spikes in a neuron have no encoded image information. That defective vision is not due to spike codes, but like astigmatism or myopia, is anatomical, suggests that spikes simply and robustly move z location, in which image x-y resolution is due to receptor spacing and diameter.

Single retinal receptors sense a small area; subsequent RFs integrate in stages so that the largest cortical RF matches emergent spatial perceptions with receptor image resolution. But for monocular RFs to integrate binocularly, a graduated anatomical matching requires a divergence to finer, alternating monocular strips in cortex.[40] First, the optic nerve,

---

[38] RGC's adapt over time to any stimulus intensity within the orders of magnitudes possible, effectively rescaling their response so that a greatly limited spike output range results. This similar output to a wide input range is an ambiguous information code however--see Baccus, S. & Meister, M. (2002) Neuron $\underline{36}$:909 (discussed further in the last chapter of this book). Power-matching requires spike output to self-limit when input photons are so excessive that they saturate receptor capacity; see French, op. cit. Since just one spike is necessary to move z-axis location of an unchanging stimulus amplitude, adaptation that limits spike output makes parsimonious sense.

[39] Yellott, J., Wandell, B., Cornsweet, T. (1984) Handbook of Sensory Physiology (Geiger, S. ed.) Sec.1; $\underline{3}$:257.

[40] Hubel, D. & Weisel, T. (1977) Proc. Roy. Soc. Lon. $\underline{198}$:1, first gave evidence of a hierarchy of anatomical stages: a course monocular input parses into bilaterally organized visual fields at LGN and subdivides to a finer scale of monocular strips, which integrate the retinal visual fields binocularly in V1 and V2 cortex.

termed the optic tract (OT) after splitting, crosses so that the visual field in each eye divides: the right halves of the two retinas go to the left LGN, and the left halves to the right. The left hemifields from both eyes alternate layers in the right LGN, similarly for the left LGN, so that the total of six layers in the LGN are constituted of four contiguous P layers and two layers of M input, all in retinotopic register with the external visual field.[41]

The LGN and its complex circuitry are an intermediate step for the graduated retinotopic match of the same halves of the visual field from each eye into adjacent V1 strips, which then converge to binocular synapses in areas V1 and V2.[42] The retinotopic alignment of six layers in each LGN, allows an x-y match of locations in the image during fixation, so that the succession of z spikes corresponding to any retinal location, fuse into a temporal continuum.[43]

At first glance, synapses that reduce average spike rates at LGN can be interpreted as an impedance mismatch of the progressive increase in RF areas. However, the equal numbers of RGC and LGN neurons, and the close match of the circular diameters of LGN RFs with RGC RFs, from the right and left retinas that overlap in LGN RFs covering the same half of the visual field, also corresponds with a halv-

---

[41] See Sincich, L. & Horton, J. (2005) Ann. Rev. Neurosci. $\underline{28}$:303, to review the details of this primate visual anatomy.

[42] To clarify: the complexity of synaptic connectivity in LGN is an underlying anatomical structure that supports overlying transfer of the z-location of an image edge, without reconstructing imagery itself.

[43] As will be discussed in Chapter Three, movies empirically set at 24 frames/sec, integrate sequentially at the same retinotopically invariant map, so that smooth motion over time, rather than a blur, or a strobe, is sensed. This z fusion of x-y frames must occur early in the visual pathway, most likely in the six overlapping maps in each LGN.

ing of stimulated spike rate.[44] This reduced spike rate makes sense if the LGN aligns six layers of x-y locations by spatial overlap, without increasing RF areas. The precise retinotopic alignment of two P layers from each eye at each x-y location, can reduce z spike output by a third, due to the redundancy of the four total P layers, while also increasing output spike reliability. The precise alignment of repeated LGN x-y layers means that x-y information in labeled neurons is not coded by reduced LGN spike rates. Here, spikes move *only* the z location over time, *not* detailed x-y data; neurons that traverse retinotopic maps move identical z spikes; x-y dimensions are solely determined by the map. Subsequent stages increase spatial convergence and divergence of neurons without encoding additional x-y labeled information into z spikes. The increase in serial RF areas that correlates with increased neural distance from the retina and reduced spike rates, constitutes a biological impedance match system.[45]

Output from the bilateral LGN, each with input from both retinas covering half of the visual field, is termed the optic radiation (OR), which diverges into alternating strips from each eye on the surface of the two hemispheric cortices, which is an impedance match of the dual monocular visual fields by contiguous alternating strips. The binocular juxtaposi-

---

[44] Carandini, M., Horton, J., Sincich, L. (2007) J. Vision 7:20.1; Spear, P., Kim, C., Ahmad, A., Tom, B. (1996) Vis. Neurosci. 13:199; Usrey et al., op. cit.; Sincich, L., Horton, J., Sharpee, T. (2009) J. Neurosci. 29:6207. Halved spike rates at LGN, and similar diameters of RGC and LGN RFs, are robust findings in cats and primates. Postsynaptic temporal summation, with no spatial summation, halves rates for spike z fusion in the aligned LGN RF. The closer spike pairs occur, the more likely that the last stimulates a reemitted spike.

[45] See other biological analogs of impedance matching in French, op. cit. An impedance match plot is shown later in this chapter in *Fig. 5*.

tion enables synapses to converge a binocular perception of the image. The alternating monocular strips interweave orthogonally with bands of retinotopic large V1/V2 RFs, each with radial simple cells that respond to all orientations of stimulus edges.

P neurons input into the bottom of layer 4C in primate V1; these, along with M input, converge onto simple cells in V1 upper layers, to create directionally oriented RFs.[46] Simple cells are thought to detect features to reconstruct the V1 image, but V1 awareness of retinal resolution must be via the reiteration of the foveal map by P cells, which occupy the hub in the center of the radially oriented simple cell RFs.[47] The simple cell RF responds to oriented edge length resulting from convergence of multiple aligned RGC RFs, in which the simple cell reemits highest rates to the aligned retinal feature.[48] Simple cell RFs converge in turn into complex cell RFs.[49]

---

[46] The ovally symmetric simple cell RFs respond at highest spike rates to a narrow bar, of specific orientation and a length several times its width, moving at an optimal rate and direction; in Hubel, D. & Wiesel, T. (1962) J. Physiol. 160:106. This description of simple cell orientation selectivity in higher mammals is to indicate that successive cortical areas of synaptic convergence, match increasingly complex feature synthesis from labeled retinal receptor patterns. To examine a cortical map of labeled lines, see Chklovskii et al., op. cit.

[47] Macaque oriented V1 RFs in layers 2-3, also known as simple cells, respond 10 msec after initial layer 4C response, peaking in magnitude 60 msec later; in Lund, J., Angelucci, A., Bressloff, P. (2003) Cereb. Cort. 13:15. Described further in Chap. Three, macaques, in contrast to cats, have V1 P cells with small RFs, which occupy the central blob of radially arranged simple cells with oriented RFs; in Latawiec, D., Martin, K., Meskenaite, V. (2000) J. Comp. Neurol. 419:306 and Sincich, L. & Horton, J. (2005) Ann. Rev. Neurosci. 28:303.

[48] It is also necessary to parse motion into oriented directions in all parts of V1, to filter directional signals to V5 cortex, which then can sense directional motion in all parts of the visual field.

[49] Anzai, A., Peng, X., Van Essen, D. (2007) Nature Neurosci. 10:1313.

Complex cells respond to angles from all directions, correlating with the percept of perspective.[50] In V4 cortex, further RF convergence responds to more complex shapes and slant in three dimensions.[51]

The 12% of total RGCs in the central 4 degrees of fovea that retinotopically map to 27% of the surface area of V1 cortex, is consistent with a ~100:1 increase in V1 cell numbers per cone.[52] However, this ratio may also explain why less than 10% of V1 excitatory synapses are from LGN inputs.[53] The convolutions on visual cortex, the sulci and gyri, magnify cortical surface area relative to the retinal surface. P neurons predominate as input to expanded foveal V1 RFs.[54] Expansion of upper layers of V1 cortex accommodates more interneurons and convergence and divergence to more neurons and synapses, which reemit at lower rates than their inputs. Total V1 neurons in primates outnumber input LGN neurons by more than 100:1 and V1 cells reemit

---

[50] Does neural convergence reiterate the convergence of perspective? Euclid's fifth postulate states that parallel lines do not meet, but does not distinguish convergent perspective from the actual fan-like convergence of lines to a point. Curiously, the Greeks used a curvilinear perspective to construct buildings, so that they would be perceived to have straight lines. See Optics, Painting & Photography (1970), by Pirenne, M., pp. 148, 181 for discussion and primary references.

[51] Hinkle, D. & Connor, C. (2002) Nature Neurosci. 5:665.

[52] Wikler, K., Williams, R., Rakic, P. (1990) J. Comp. Neurol. 297: 499; Suner, I. & Rakic, P. (1996) Vis. Neurosci. 13:586.

[53] Adams, D. & Horton, J. (2003) J. Neurosci. 23:3771, Peters et al., op. cit.; only 2-8% of excitatory synapses in V1 are from LGN; the majority of V1 excitatory synapses are from other visual areas.

[54] Hubel, D. & Wiesel,T. (1974) J. Comp. Neurol. 158:295; Schein, S. & de Monasterio, F. (1987) J. Neurosci. 7:996. P neurons/degree of visual arc, and the cortical surface area/degree of visual arc, are highest in foveal cortex. The number of M neurons/cortical surface area, compared to the P ratio, increases greatly in peripheral cortex.

less than half the LGN cell rate.[55] So, are spikes a sparse temporal code to reconstruct a V1 image? Spatial linearity is not distorted because the larger foveal RFs in V1 cortex are centered on the same retinotopic x-y locations as cone RFs.[56]

This difference in neural granularity between retinal and larger cortical RFs raises the question of how fixational movements of retinal RFs are translated into spikes on the z axis of the optic nerve, OT and LGN radiations. For the P system, this has to be a function of the edges of receptor RFs, which can be stimulated by typical tremor amplitudes. Retinal tremor, in humans with dominant frequencies in the range of 60-100 Hz, averaging about 80 Hz,[57] stimulates spikes at high rates from midget RGCs.[58] FEMs that span a longer distance, drifts and microsaccades, are sized for larger RFs in V1 cortex. High

---

[55] Stevens. C. (2001) Nature 422:39; Briggs, F. & Usrey, W. (2007) Front. Integr. Neurosci. 1:3; Alonso, J., Usrey, W., Reid, R. (2001) J. Neurosci. 21:4002; Babadi, B. & Sompolinsky, H. (2014) Neuron 83:1213.

[56] Kara & Reid, op. cit.; precise superposition of V1 RFs and RGC RFs occurs despite cat and primate differences in divergence from RGCs to LGN and from LGN to V1, detailed in Peters et al., op. cit.

[57] Martinez-Conde et al., op. cit.; McCamy, M., Collins, N., Otero-Millan J., Al-Kallani, M., Macknik, S., Coakley, D., Troncoso, X., Boyle, G., Narayanan, V., Wolfe, T., Martinez-Conde, S. (2013) Peer J. 1:e14; Eizenman, M., Hallett, P., Frecker, R. (1985) Vis. Res. 25:1635. V1 sustained neurons respond better to drifts, while V1 phasic neurons respond preferentially to microsaccades. Both types of fixational movements cover a distance at least a dozen times greater in length than a cone's diameter. The Troxler effect suggests that tremor amplitudes can sustain spikes from small cone RF edges, but cannot sustain spikes from the parasol-like M RGC RFs in peripheral retina.

[58] Greschner, M., Bongard, M., Rujan, P., Ammermuller, J. (2002) Nature Neurosci. 5:341, show that slow 5 Hz tremor in turtles (spanning the RGC RF width) doubles individual and population sustained spike rates compared to the stationary retinal condition, under constant light conditions; turtle retina is evolutionarily very similar to human.

RGC spike rates could possibly be a temporal code to overcome the receptor to RGC spatial bottleneck (except at foveola); V1 cells, which diverge with no bottleneck, serially reduce rates except at high stimulus frequencies that rapidly reemit.[59]

Hyperacuity, the ability to detect the location of minimal stimuli, is much better than spatial resolution resolvable by the diameter and spacing of the smallest foveal cones.[60] The location of gaps in edges of simple stimuli can be detected easily by experimental subjects, but easily confounds with edge contrast and the resolution measured for contoured line stimuli. It is thought that the constant drifts, tremor and microsaccades that shift the retinal receptors, provoke potentials in the plexiform layers that get translated into a sustained complex code in RGCs, which in cortex, are processed statistically over time. An alternative view espoused here, is that spikes move z locations of the foveal x-y map to the fine neural grain in larger cortical RFs, where increased numbers of synapses for the same x-y location fire in response to the temporal and spatial convergence of input spikes. Perceived hyperacuity results because retinal tremor initiates

---

[59] Briggs & Usrey, op. cit.; LGN cells stimulated at 30-40 Hz reemit to and from directly connected V1 cells at similar frequencies, due to temporal facilitation at synapses.

[60] See Westheimer (1979) Investig. Opthalm. Vis. Sci. $\underline{18}$:892; vernier hyperacuity detects less than 10 sec of arc of offset of bar stimuli, finer than the resolution of adjacent point stimuli by contiguous foveal cones spaced at ~30 sec of visual arc. The smallest foveal cones in humans are about 1.3 microns in diameter, with center-to center spacing of 2.5 microns, in Ahnelt, P. (1998) Eye $\underline{12}$:531. To compare with foveal resolution, smaller V1 RFs span about .2 degrees, or 12 minutes of visual arc at one degree of foveal eccentricity (Hubel & Wiesel, 1974, op. cit.). The alternative measures of resolving power--visual angle of arc vs. cone diameter and spacing, are discussed in Schein et al., op. cit.

spikes with a great receptor-edge precision vis-a-vis the position of a stimulus edge than is evident from receptor spacing; a spike emits repeatably from an edge as it moves across a receptor RF boundary.[61]

The overlap of monocular x-y locations at binocular neurons, at the same time, also makes disparity based discriminations that are better than hyperacuity. This stereoacuity[62] results because binocularly driven synapses in V1 and V2, sense disparity via temporally synchronous convergent spikes that re-emit perceptual spikes from monocularly aligned inputs.[63] 3D stereovision is sensed only when monocular locations emit synchronously, then reemit from x-y aligned binocular synapses. It may not be that broad tuning of neurons collectively codes stereoacuity; spikes emitted abruptly at the same edge in each retina, match latencies precisely at retinotopically aligned binocular neurons, which rapidly reemit to perceptually endure as stereovision.

The feature or percept of x-y 'length', here, converges from linearly arranged retinal receptors that spatially summate ultimately to V1 oriented simple cell RFs. The spike intervals or rate do not code oriented edge length; rather simultaneously stimulated receptors, at an equal distance to a spatially convergent neuron, synchronously stimulate an onward

---

[61] Greschner, et al., op. cit.

[62] Westheimer, G. (1994) Proc. Roy. Soc. London B <u>257</u>:205.

[63] Read, J. & Cumming, B. (2005) J. Neurophys. <u>94</u>:1541, discuss the implications of interocular spike delays of a few milliseconds to visual cortex, for sensing spatial disparity of monocular images and resultant stereoacuity. Westheimer & McKee, op. cit., find that stereoacuity is highest in the fixational plane, even though the retinal images may shift 1-3 min of arc during fixation; stereoacuity, which depends on the precise relative disparity of a single image point in the monocular images, has a much smaller deviation of 3-6 sec of arc.

spike. Z spikes themselves, here do not code x-y edge length, so the percept or awareness of linear orientation is not confounded by variable spike noise or spike rates. Neurons have a length and route necessary to connect sensory arrays with cortical locations, but this variable anatomy is also not sensed or coded by spikes. As defined here, any 1D z-axis traverses repeated x-y surfaces without encoding 2D image or surface dimensions.[64] The repetition of 2D surfaces in embryonic development,[65] creates the equal paths for spikes that temporally synchronize at retinotopically aligned, spatially convergent synapses. FEM-generated identical spikes at the retinas do not encode shifting x-y image information but synchronize at binocular neurons in V1/V2 areas to create an unshifting, 3D x-y-z stable stereoscopic feature awareness, due to the emitted and reemitted perceptual synchrony of proximal-distal 1D z spikes, as will be described in more detail.

Experimental paradigms that assume cell spike rate is a 1D temporal code of data, do not agree with the alternative concept here that spikes move 1D z locations across topographic 2D arrays. While a spatial frequency of 60 cycles/degree stimulates a high rate

---

[64] Emergent cognitive processes tell us that length on the axon's z axis adds, but repeated subunits do not create length, as judged by a primary entity such as an AP, which does not encode the addition. Thus for repetitive, identical spikes, the V1 retinotopic map cannot be differentiated by its z distance from the retina, despite the spike latencies that observers impose as an accumulative property.

[65] Wedeen, V., Rosene, D., Wang, R., Dai, G., Mortazavi, F., Hagmann, P., Kaas, J., Tseng, W-Y. (2012) Science 335:1628; rather than complex 3D cortical structures, advanced anatomical analysis shows grids of neurons organized as repeated 2D surfaces similar to those in the brainstem. It is shown that cortical maps are repeated 2D surfaces, not connected as 3D spirals; repeated topography results from a sequential embryonic process. Mathematically, it is improbable that two families of 3D curves can orient to have a common 2D surface; rather, a 2D surface forms initially and replicates in 3D space and time.

of primate foveal spikes above background rate, cortical or behaviorally measured spatial resolution is somewhat lower. If one bypasses the eye's optics with laser interference fringes on the retina, LGN neurons fire (above background rate) at 120 cycles/degree.[66] So with this capacity for high spatial resolution, why is an exogenous 60 cycles/degree detected as a lower spatial frequency in the LGN and cortex? Spatial frequency gratings generate reduced AP cortical rates, compared to retinal rates, due to greater spatial and temporal integration in higher order neurons. Here, the concept that spikes move z locations orthogonal to neural arrays, suggests also that a neuron's frequency response is not a data code but an epiphenomenon of the integration area of an RF. The stimulation of spike rates by defined spatial frequencies, can be called an artifact due to the spectrum of response by any large collection of neurons to any imposed stimulus. As stated, reduced cortical spike rates from successive synaptic integrations are not sparsely coding image resolution. Here 1D spikes transfer z location from the retina across 2D arrays, which retinotopically reiterate foveola resolution via temporal summation, rather than as spatial x-y data in a temporal code.

That every neuron responds at highest spike rate to its best stimulating spatial frequency, can as an averaged population, code a specific spatial frequency,[67] is actually evidence for the idea that diverse response rates in a neural population mean at least one neuron responds to any stimulus frequency. The overlapped tuning of a collection of neurons,

---

[66] McMahon, M., Lahkneet, M., Lennie, P., Williams, D. (2000) J. Neurosci. 20:2043.

[67] De Valois, R., Albrecht, D., Thorell, L. (1982) Vis. Res. 22:545.

impedance matches by responding to the total range of contrasts in natural scenes.[68] Neurons perturbed at specific frequencies have varied spiking responses, but z spikes here, emitted by RGC types that respond to features, are identical within the RGC anatomical and feature labels. A color-labeled foveal cone stimulates On and Off and P or M RGC types that may overlap its RF; a majority of these RGC types produce spikes from that one cone. A perifoveal RGC also produces similar spike responses to any cone type in its RF, if the cone's input strength is accounted for.[69] This data directly supports the assertion here that the anatomy is the x-y labeled code, not the z spikes. The variable spike rates in many neurons to a single stimulus, are a location and intensity population response, not a repeatably defined code.

Stimulation from x-y locations at the skin maps to equivalent topographic locations on repeated somatotopic maps; this constraint transfers only z location by spikes, the x-y information is reiterated in topographically aligned RFs. This is apparent phenomenologically in that touch that stimulates spikes is felt at the skin, even though the spike terminus is in perceptual cortex. In contrast, stimulated cortical activity that does not result from labeled receptor input, generates only an ambiguous feeling of a phantom limb.[70] The high resolution foveola, in con-

---

[68] Laughlin, S. (1981) Z. Naturforsch. C 36:910; response to varying input was recorded from large monopolar (bipolar) cells of fly retina.

[69] Li, P., Field, G., Greschner, M., Ahn, D., Gunning, D., Mathieson, K., Sher, A., Litke, A., Chichilnisky, E. (2014) Neuron 81:130; that a perifoveal RGC responds to any cone type in its RF is called univariance; 'input strength' is a term that relates the distance of the stimulated cone from the RGC center, including contrast and response kinetics.

[70] Pereira, J. & Alves, R. (2011) Medical Hypotheses 77:853.

trast to the perifovea mentioned in the last paragraph, preserves peripheral x-y label specificity because the dominant input to a midget RGC is from one cone.[71] An abrupt spike response to edge contrast, and increased rate with stimulus intensity, has no x-y information, but identical z spikes through reiterated 2D maps, move to equivalent x-y locations in V1 cortex, to temporally correlate cortical x-y retinotopy with receptor x-y locations.

The auditory system, like the somatosensory system, responds collectively to a specific sound via the initial impedance matched responses of specific inner hair cells (IHC) in the cochlea of the inner ear. Each IHC contacts a few to 20 spiral ganglion neurons (SGNs). Each SGN responds with a different threshold and range of spike rate, to the loudness of the characteristic frequency at which the IHC fires maximally. A price of low SGN threshold is that many spikes are spontaneously generated that are not evoked by a specific frequency. This noise is not perceived; rather, these noisy spikes are filtered out because they do not converge in synchrony at synapses. But impedance matching in multiple SGNs requires a response at any frequency and intensity; as intensity increases, SGNs with higher thresholds

---

[71] Demb, J. & Brainard, D. (2010) Nature 467:670, point out that one midget RGC connects to one foveal cone (which divides to an Off and an On midget RGC via bipolar cells) to keep the cone type color specific. Field, G., Gauthier, J., Sher, A., Greschner, M., Machado, T., Jepson, L., Shlens, J., Gunning, D., Mathieson, K., Dabrowski, W., Paninski, L., Litke, A., Chichilnisky, E. (2010) Nature 467:673, show that perifoveal RGCs emit spikes preferably from the dominant cone type closest to the RF center. In the fovea, one cone dominates the input to a midget RGC, with color opponent inputs in the surround, so that an RGC does not transmit hue as a multiplexed code. Field, G., Sher, A., Gauthier, J., Greschner, M., Shlens, J., Litke, A., Chichilnisky, E. (2007) J. Neurosci. 27:13261, show that opposing On and Off midget RGCs are in separate plexiform layers and labeled lines, with faster, more sustained On center than Off center responses.

are recruited. While loud sounds induce deafness, in IHCs this loudness broadens tuning, which adds noisy spikes to the spike rates of SGNs.[72]

A sound frequency at the outer range of IHC sensitivity, stimulates a lower spike frequency from the SGN. For example, at 4 kHz (humans hear up to 24 kHz), an IHC may have a maximal response rate just in this range; but a contacting SGN may have an initial response that peaks at 1 kHz, which quickly adapts to a lower rate of 400 spikes/sec.[73]

These data show that spike rates coincide with sound frequency reliably only at very low frequencies. At higher sound frequencies, SGN spikes respond precisely to the same phase of the stimulus frequency cycle, skipping a predictable number of cycles before spiking at the same phase of the frequency cycle. It is somewhat counterintuitive that SGN spike rates have a dynamic range that is a fraction of the range of frequencies perceived; tonotopic mapping in auditory cortex, which correspond to the frequency order of IHCs in the cochlea, allows an accurate perception of sound frequencies rather than of spike rates. As mentioned, deaf-inducing noise damages receptors, IHCs and connected synapses, which degenerate to cause a peripheral loss of sensation; this loss may be due to more noise but not to lower SGN or cortical spike rates. So sound perception is not a direct spike frequency or rate.

To repeat, the correspondence of a point on the cochlea of the inner ear to a location on a cortical

---

[72] Henry, K. & Heinz, M. (2012) Nature Neurosci. 15:1362.

[73] Buran, B., Stvenzke, N., Neef, A., Gundelfinger, E., Moser, T., Liberman, M.C. (2010) J. Neurosci. 30:7587; Palmer, A. & Russell, I. (1986) Hear. Res. 24:1.

map is an anatomical 'code' of sound frequency, not spike intervals or rate. Also, spike rates that follow low or initial sound frequencies, confound with spike rate that increases with loudness; both combine in the perception of pitch, which won't be discussed here. While one neuron's spikes are not a code, the bilateral convergent timing of spikes at specific synapses reemit to locate sounds in perceptual space.[74] So temporally synchronized spikes at spatially convergent synapses result in latent perceptions.

Changes in tone are signaled by temporally precise compound action potentials and initial high spike rates in responsive SGNs. Contrast in tone in IHCs (and in light in retinal cells) are signaled by abrupt, quantitative releases of vesicles from ribbons inside the pre-synaptic ending of the neuron; the abrupt post-synaptic change in spike rate signals the abrupt contrast that signals the initial time of sensation.[75] The abrupt spikes, along with rate that is proportional to intensity, synchronously summate at convergent synapses to reemit perceptual spikes.

The outlined somatotopic and auditory sensory systems, as with the visual system, integrate perceptions in succeeding larger RFs via precise temporal convergence of spikes from multiple receptors. Increased cortical area, for example, can accommodate more musical inputs, to fine-tune synaptic firing to coincident APs, so that motor cortex can coordinate the dexterity of musical performance. The

---

[74] Proctor, L. & Konishi, M. (1997) PNAS (USA) 16:10421. Timing codes have also evolved over time in other systems; see Carr. C., Amagai, S., Kubke, M., Massoglia, D. (1996) Proc. 24th Gottingen Neurobiol. Conf. p. 83.

[75] LoGuidice, L. & Matthews, G. (2009) Neuroscientist 15:380; the synaptic ribbons act as scaffolds so that with abrupt stimulation, many vesicles release at the same time into the synaptic cleft.

term 'code' is more useful to indicate that a sensory spatio-temporal spike pattern generates in a population of motor neurons, spikes that sequence a precisely timed motor pattern.[76]

For flickering flashes of light, the fovea's P neurons respond more slowly than the M system that predominates in the periphery of the retina, which follows flicker with better temporal resolution at higher frequencies. A learned, repeatable temporal spike code for imagery would have to reliably predict each of the multitude of visual objects it is possible to sense, and code for similar but never-before-seen stimuli. While retinal receptors respond to flicker at temporal frequencies up to 120 Hz, fusion in foveal horizontal cells of the retinal plexus occurs at about 60 Hz in humans, which is also the perceptual threshold; this smearing of graded potentials in the plexiform layers of the retina is a major factor in perceptual blur.[77] In addition, spatially diffuse flicker of 60 Hz or higher frequencies, is integrated at successive synapses to be perceived as blur in cortex. But retinal tremor at 80 Hz that is a blur to the external observer, shifts high-contrast image edges across the boundaries of foveal receptors. This peripheral temporal resolution is preserved by tremor-timed spikes that temporally synchronize at LGN and V1 convergent synapses, to result in sharp

---

[76] Olveczky, B., Otchy, T., Goldberg, J., Aranov, D., Fee, M. (2011) J. Neurophys. 106:386.

[77] Fusion frequency depends on many factors, such as stimulus area, intensity, and retinal location, reviewed in Van de Grind, W.A., Grusser, O.-J., Lunkenheimer, H.-U. (1973) Handbook of Sensory Physiology, 7:3A (Jung, R., ed.). They document the successive reduction in range of average firing rates from RGCs to V2 cortex, in response to a constant flicker rate. Above about 60 Hz, flicker is perceived as a fused blur because the whole retina averages graded potentials over repeated flicker cycles to generate fewer spikes.

cortical perceptions of a shifting image, which should lack resolution if temporally and spatially summated at each serially convergent synapse. One cannot diminish the importance of experiments that show that a stimulus edge across a cone boundary, reliably causes a spatially and temporally precise spike to emit from its RGC.[78] Small cortical pyramidal cell circuits generate gamma rhythms (30-100 Hz), which may stimulate oculomotor muscles and their tremor rates.[79] Thalamo-cortical oscillations, synchronizing with tremor, can be interpreted as a temporal code that is decoded in cortex.[80] However as will be shown, edge-generated spikes do not temporally code information to reconstruct imagery in cortex, but as moving z locations, synchronize cortical perception with retinal information.

One must differentiate the temporal frequency of stimulus flicker from physiological tremor rate: at low exogenous flash flicker frequencies, the average cell spike rate of foveal RGCs coincides with flicker rate--but as flicker increases to higher frequencies, spikes fire for every other flash, then every fourth flash, then at flicker fusion, diminish to a much lower maintained rate.[81] If spikes move only the retinal z location of stimuli, then uniform visual field flicker stimulation of the plexiform layers, needs few RGC spikes to transmit the temporally unvarying fusion of plexiform potentials. The decline of the per-

---

[78] Greschner et al., op. cit.; For turtles, tremor amplitude that is less than the width of the photoreceptor is less likely to elicit a spike.

[79] Buzsaki, G., Logothetis, N., Singer, W. (2013) Neuron 80:751; Eizenman et al., op. cit; or does tremor causes gamma rhythms?

[80] This model is in Ahissar, E. & Arieli, A. (2001) Neuron 32:185.

[81] Crevier, D. & Meister, M. (1998) J. Neurophys 79:1869.

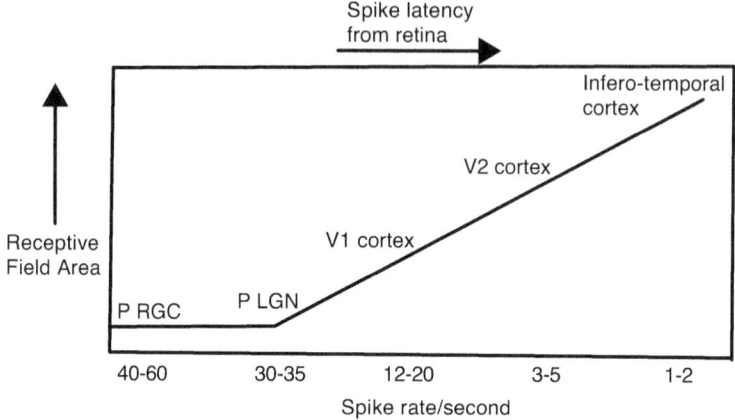

Fig. 5: This graph illustrates the rule that light flicker at the retina causes average neuronal firing rate to decline proportionally, or impedance match, at each synaptic stage (Van de Grind et al., op. cit.). RF areas in primates increase serially by a factor of about 2.5 from the LGN stage onwards (Rolls, E. (2000) Neuron 27:205); spike latency also increases with the neuronal length to each stage (Capalbo, M., Postma, E., Goebel R. (2008) PLoS Comp. Biol. 4:e1000159; Hung et al., op. cit. Chapter Three). Data shown are from cats and primates that scale invariantly even though brain size differs (Eytan, D. & Marom, S. (2006) J. Neurosci. 26:8465; Buzsaki et al., op. cit.). The arbitrary units of this characteristic curve may shift, depending on specific experimental conditions.

ceived flicker rate (when stimulation is higher than 3 Hz, convergent spike rates at subsequent cortical perceptual areas are lower than spike rate at V1)[82], shows that spikes that transfer z location of the exogenous image to later cortical areas, are firing and being perceived at a lower temporal frequency than

---

[82] Van de Grind et al., op. cit., pp. 462-485. Above the flicker fusion rate, On-center neurons sustain at a rate identical to that imposed by a flicker stimulus of the same luminance, while Off-center neurons, responding to the part of the flicker cycle with no light, reduce response duration. The separation of overlapping Off and On systems initiated at bipolar cells is retained in expanded cortical RFs; mutually inhibitory types of On- and Off-center neurons respond reciprocally to the presence and absence of light so that z location at a single cone is transmitted centrally on separate pathways via reciprocal firing rates, without being a multiplexed code in a single neuron.

that of the exogenous flicker modulation (*Fig. 5*). These cumulative synaptic area summations are due to spatially diffuse flicker that is not as spatially and temporally precise as edge contrast-sensitive tremor-generated spikes at RGC and LGN synapses.

The serial reduction of high RGC spike rates to lower average neuronal spike rates in cortical stages that succeed V1 cortex, shows that cognition of stimulus flicker rate does not jibe with the high temporal and spatial precision of RGC spikes. The cognitive cortical neurons count the collective spike firing at a lower average rate, due to previous stages of synaptic summations. While some V1 M neurons may respond veridically to high foveal flicker rates, the sustained response of multitudinous P cells reemit into a dominant if delayed cortical perception, and temporally converge the large spatial scale of higher retinal flicker rates, to a lower perceived cortical z spike rate with longer intervals between spikes.

This chapter has described a process that impedance matches external image stimulation through the repeated retinotopic arrays of the visual system. The information in the image is not coded by spikes to be cortically decoded, instead photons emitted or reflected from a location in physical space stimulate the retinal emission of spikes, defined here as z locations, which move through repeated retinotopic x-y surfaces. Due to the repetition of topographically aligned arrays along parallel z axes, the distributed, moving locations of z spikes in neurons do not aggregate quantitatively, as reasoned earlier, so are z equivalent. However, the accompanying increase in RF area, from the retina to cortex, impedance matches external image space with the visual brain's increased numbers of convergent synapses in larger RFs, finally creating a full perception and increased awareness, or repetitive z consciousness, of external dimensions and imagery. An important consequence of this impedance match of graduated 2D RF areas via movement of z spikes, is that the cortical reiteration of an unshifting external image via decoding of shifting retinal information is not required.

CONCLUSIONS

We invoke several rules to reinterpret the function of neuronal spikes:

1) A spike is a spatial location that moves along the length of the neuron. Multiple spikes of a sustained character are identical z locations, distributed along any topographically aligned route through connected neurons.

2) The external image plane shifts at the proximal, anatomically fixed sensory surface. The fixational shifting of the retinal x-y plane stimulates spikes on each RGC z axis. The spikes issuing at distal synaptic arrays compete with other parallel z inputs to keep that retinotopic array topographically aligned with the proximal end.

3) The unchanging quality of the AP as it traverses the length of any neuron, indicates that z distance in the neuron is not aggregated or coded by the z spike. X-y dimensional properties are unvarying at any position along the z axis of any topographically aligned neuron. The concept of z equivalence at repeated, retinotopically aligned 2D surfaces makes explicit the lack of x-y temporal coding by z spikes.

4) The identical nature of spikes in labeled neurons, means only the intensity and timing of spikes are conveyed to convergent synapses, where temporal and spatial summation cause fewer onward spikes to emit. This change in spike location in aligned neurons, displaces the z coordinate of the retinal image rather than temporally coding image information to reconstruct the image cortically.

Sequential Conscious Time and Symmetry

When afferent sensations change location to 'higher cortical centers', the perception at these centers is that the decision to move, for example, an arm, is occurring consciously in real time in response to peripheral sensations. So while cortical decisions take time to respond to sensory information from the periphery, somehow this conscious decision-making doesn't seem delayed. While the z equivalence hypothesis may be shown to play a role in the slow perception of rapid sensory events, a decision making process based on timely peripheral sensations requires a reversal of the usual cause-effect sequence for the brain to 'know' it is responding quickly as unpredictable exogenous events occur.

The normal cause of cortical events is stimulation at the sensory periphery. The initial spikes at the periphery will be stated as "0" in time; by the time the APs from this peripheral event have traversed several orders of neurons, the cortical time for consciousness and the accompanying decision-making process have taken up several hundred milliseconds, as measured with the time course of evoked potentials on the cortical surface. This is consistent with the experimental finding that about 250 milliseconds of cortical electrode stimulation is necessary for the observer to sense that the stimulation time coincides with the consciousness resulting from natural peripheral sensation; cortical conscious sensation occurs much more quickly with direct skin stimulation that lasts at least 30 msec.[83] The next chapter analyzes in vision, how sustained spikes present in cortical somatotopic areas before the 30 msec skin stimulation, shifts the normally delayed perception to the skin stimulation very quickly.

Other experiments of this type show that when the brain wills a finger movement, it becomes conscious of its intention after a neurophysiological indicator, the Readiness Potential, a recorded signal from many neurons that is an indicator of impending finger movement, has already passed. Similarly to sensation initiated at the skin, the cortex, in order to feel that it is in conscious control of events in real time, creates "0" time as the conscious cortical time, rather than the prior Readiness Potential. The motor movement occurs with an objective delay of about 220 msec after one is conscious of willing the movement; also, the actual time that one moves the finger is 60-80 msec later than one is conscious of moving the finger (as measured visually on a rotating clockface by Libet's subject). By reversing time, so that delayed conscious sensation is actually

---

[83] Libet, B., Wright, E., Feinstein, B., Pearl, D. (1979) Brain 194:191; Libet, B., Wright, E., Gleason, C. (1982) Electoenceph. and Clin. Neurophys. 54:322. Sensation by cortical stimulation may be delayed due to orthodromic resistance that takes a much longer time than the sustained spike train that coincides in time at skin and cortex when skin is stimulated for 30 msec.

"0" in time, rather than the initial Readiness Potential or a skin stimulus as the initial time, all other neural events are now relative to this conscious "0" time. What conventional logic says are earlier events, now proceed in a positive time direction from this delayed conscious time, so that the brain's consciousness of its delayed reaction (to peripheral sensation or motor activation) is reversed without being paradoxical or invoking a negative time direction.

A simple model can be created to reflect that time has to be "reversed" for conscious decision-making to be perceived as being in a positive time direction. Initial spikes from the periphery at time "0" reach the cognitive center still bearing this time "0" tag, but with a delay of say "4" from the initial peripheral stimulation. Given, the conscious cortex thinks it is "0" in time, and by much cogitation, that the peripheral receptor responds to the same sensation earlier in time. To the cortex, this represents an earlier event, in that initial time has shifted from the peripheral sensation at 0 time to the cortical knowledge of that sensation, which is the new 0 time. Cortical consciousness therefore has no sense that it is delayed at time "0", and certainly has no sense that this time has gone past the previous conscious point in time, since no consciousness of the future exists before time sequences into the future. The essence of conscious sensation is that it is always on time, that it is "0" in time, as conventional time passes sequentially. *Fig. 2.1* illustrates the notion that "0" is cortical consciousness in real time; the conscious "now" has no sense of latency (or sense of sequential time) as it steps through 0-0-0-0-0-0.

A sense of latency results from cycling through via the numerical sequence shown (0-1-2-3-4) to another anatomical site, such as the LGN (vision) or the ventroposterolateral nuclei (VPL, touch) of the thalamus. These numbers represent time to conscious cortex as an anatomically distant location rather than an abstract duration which may not be comprehended by single neurons; reified "time" to the brain's conscious real-time processing has to be realized as a spatially defined neuronal locus.[84] Conscious sensation is a necessary condition before any sense of time as memory can be established.

```
Cyclical sequence:      0
                        1 0
                        2 1 0
                        3 2 1 0
                        4 3 2 1 0
                        5 4 3 2 1 0
Externally defined sequence:      -1 0 1
```

Fig. 2.1: Model of time reversal from conscious sense of "0" time (the instant that constitutes "now"), to distant anatomical sites. "5" represents an anatomical site, such as the LGN, which is earlier in time and distance in the neuronal chain of synaptic events. Neurons diverge from site 5 via succeeding synapses to other sites, such as V1, V2 etc. cortical areas. Consciousness is a sequence of 0 times, without memory, as shown by the diagonal sequence in the diagram; the time delay of conscious sensation from the periphery is represented quantitatively by the sequential locations labeled 5, 4, 3, 2, 1. Travel back in time, as to a memory, proceeds from conscious "0" in real-time, sequentially to older memories: 1, 2, 3, 4, 5. These numbers represent both past memory and cortical locations in a positive sequence that indicates spike latency and the concomitant distance to any anatomical location. Consciousness itself is always at "0" time, but is tied to the chain of external events, shown by the stepwise change in 0 position as external clock time passes, with -/+ directions, in the lowest row.

---

[84] Chapter 4 explores in detail, the concept of time as neural location.

By stepping sequentially through 0-1-2-3-4-5-4-3-2-1-0, a sort of working memory via sequential anatomical sites can occur, by going forward to anatomical sites to find the memory location, and proceeding, in the same direction, backward in sequence, back to a conscious 0 location.[85] Evidence exists that corticofugal fibers from V1 to the LGN may signal a "temporal afterimage", or a form of iconic or working memory, detected in the LGN for several seconds after cessation of a stimulus.[86] The hippocampus is in a convenient U-shaped structure that seems useful to step through to recall a particular time in a sequence (See *Fig. 2.2*). In fact, hippocampal 'place cells' have been found in CA1 and CA3 regions that respond to specific spatial locations in a maze.[87] While the hippocampus is most likely a central map representing locations as specific times, to recall quantities of specific memories this organ has to access specific neural locations in the temporal and frontal lobes. The high surface area of cortex that results from the folding of gyri (with fibers that follow the shape of the U fold) also can be an anatomical means to increase the quantity of sequentially accessible neural locations that represent specific past times.

The perception that consciousness is not altered from another anatomical site may result because: 1) the correction of the present conscious state,

---

[85] Since we are using numbers to symbolize anatomical location, using the same number heuristically, say '2' in the bidirectionally circular sequence in and out from the '0' initiation time, is through different arms of the angled sequence diagrammed in Fig. 2.1.

[86] Lehky, S. & Maunsell, J. (1996) Vision Res. 36:1225.

[87] For hippocampal coding of time and place sequences by neurons, see Lee, A. & Wilson, M. (2002) Neuron 36:1183; O'Keefe, J. & Dostrovsky, J. (1971) Brain Res. 34:171.

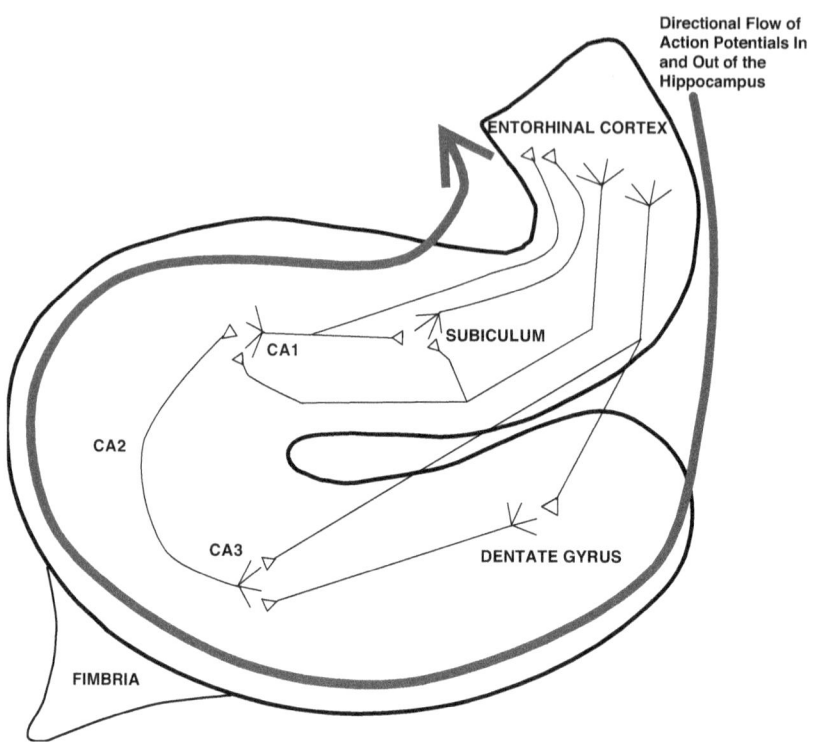

Fig. 2.2: The hippocampus is a convenient U-shaped structure that facilitates the sequential passage to and from a memory, or place, into present consciousness. Triangles signify synapses. Figure data adapted from several public sources.

via recent iconic or working memory, is via a location that becomes conscious by virtue of its transient connection to the conscious state (see *Fig. 2.1*), and 2) consciousness, by itself at any instant, is defined as having no memory, or sense of a connection to, or a retention of, its previous real-time sensation at "0". In *Fig. 2.1*, one would zigzag between layers, from 0 to 1 back to 0, to provide temporal sensation to a sensorially isolated consciousness. The cycling to a previous anatomical site like the LGN of the thalamus, or the hippocampus, constitutes a mechanism to alter the present state of consciousness by accessing an unconscious location and making it temporarily conscious. While consciousness is defined by its disconnectedness from moment to moment, not retaining any memory that would interrupt the stream of consciousness, consciousness also requires a sense of connection to a previous state in order to sense temporal continuity.

The Readiness Potential and other signals occur before conscious willing of a movement, in the Supplemental Motor Area and in frontal cortex;[88] these areas are arbitrarily named "5" of the 5-4-3-2-1-0 numbering scheme of *Fig. 2.1*. But this scheme is also consistent with the conscious volition to act at real time "0", which by definition, is always "now" and thus no event can occur after "0" in the future. One can show this play on causality in *Fig. 2.1*; if one proceeds from the first "0" at the top left down vertically to the "5" directly below, then across horizontally back to the "0"s, one would be accessing a previous state, at "5", without any lapse in sense of continuity of consciousness. While this "5" state results from a conscious *willed* volition of the perpendicular "0" state, it is a *cause* of the horizontally accessed "0" state (like a Readiness Potential causes the conscious volition to move). Being willed by, or causing consciousness, creates no contradiction, or lapsed time, to the conscious state since it retains no memory of any previous 0 state. In a reflex, movement can quickly occur before one is conscious of the sensation to do so, in that the reflexive neural circuit response is at "5" before moving to "0". In fact, consciousness is always the last effect neurally, and is always now, at "0", before any future event.

---

[88] Kornhuber, H., and Deecke, L. (1965) Pflugers Archiv 284:1; Soon, C., Brass, M., Heinze, H.-J., Haynes, J.-D. (2008) Nature Neurosci. 11:543. Is the nervous system planning unconsciously how to respond beforehand to fast events at these cortical sites? Or is it establishing synchronized neuronal activity necessary to react quickly to events as they occur? Fast reactivity is discussed in Chapter Three.

That no conscious sense of time transpires in 0-0-0-0-0-0 transitions also makes sense of the momentary lapse, or suppression, of visible sensation to consciousness during saccades (discussed in the next chapter) and eye blinks, without sensing a gap in the conscious real-time sequence 0-0-0-0-0-0 has occurred. In contrast, when one blanks out visual sensation exogenously for the same length of time as the saccade or the blink, the subject is acutely conscious of the gap in time. This is because 'time' is not consciously sensed with internal visual mechanisms, but is cognitively derived from the external shift of event to event.

The fact that one proceeds backward in time from any conscious '0' locus in *Fig. 2.1*, not a choice of directions in time, to a previous site that inputs the conscious locus, and can never step forward (into the future) from this conscious site, points to similar neural structures for accessing past memory and for imaginary meanderings "into the future" that actually are memories altering in real time.[89] Our fascination with the unpredictability of gambling expresses the reality of altering the future in real-time. Past and future are synonymous, in the same direction, to the conscious brain, and are accessed backwards and forwards from 0 time without a negative past or positive future as the 0-1-2-3-4-5-4-3-2-1-0 numerical sequence demonstrates. A neural location that symbolizes a time, which we consciously know as a memory, if strong enough, can be so intrusive as to correct the conscious, causing one to ignore peripheral sensations that intrude on imaginative images that one is attending to, as can happen to cell-phone users when driving.

---

[89] Hasssabis, D., Kumaran, D., Vann, S., Maguire, E. (2007) Proc. Nat. Acad. Sci. USA 104:1726.

The replay of memory in and out of consciousness as described with the 0-1-2-3-4-5-4-3-2-1-0 sequence in *Fig. 2.1* is shown experimentally with recordings of "ripple", which is the high frequency sequential firing of many neurons in the hippocampus. After traversing a maze, the sequence of that experience is replayed rapidly backwards by hippocampal place cells in CA1 and CA3, which were sequentially activated by locations in the maze to create memory. Before undergoing the experience again after learning, the memory is pre-played rapidly in a forward sequence. The coordinated sequence of spikes in pre-play and replay rehashes the sequential place cell locations that an animal ran through.[90] Because these neurons do not signal positive or negative directions, a sequence that proceeds backwards and forwards moves in one direction only, with time represented as neuronal locations via the single direction sequence 0-1-2-3-4-5-4-3-2-1-0. This sequential and circular time-as-location is seen also in the 'traveling wave', in which the phase of a theta (6-11 Hz) rhythm recorded at stationary electrodes progressively advances, or precesses, during the theta cycle, as recorded at any simultaneous time at sequential hippocampal locations, as theta waves are induced by the forward direction of animal travel.[91] Phase precession relates an animal's moving position with stable locations of landmarks, discussed in Chapter Four.

Whereas the location of peripheral retinal imagery is moved by z-dimension spikes on a neuron's axis,

---

[90] Diba, K. and Buzsaki, G. (2007) Nature Neuroscience 10:1241

[91] Lubenov, E.B. and Siapas, A.G. (2009) Nature 459:534, use the repeated non-reversed notation 'ABCD' to signify a circular sequence of time at place cells; the theta wave consists of oscillatory spikes within an electrode recording area that may be of various velocities.

here requiring fewer neurons and fewer action potentials than if image information was coded and transmitted, V1 cortex converges the dual x-y monocular retinal images to a single x-y binocular map. The location and timing coincidence of spikes emitted monocularly to create the perception of a stereoscopic image, is a result of spikes reemitted in V1 and V2 cortex, as discussed in the last chapter. A sort of control by perceptual attentive mechanisms in cortex, because it is at "0" time, can affect volumes of monocular spikes to cortex by acting on input that is still subconscious. Conflict of synapses altered by memories, with current spike inputs is avoided because x-y memory locations are orthogonal to moving z locations. As shown in *Fig. 2.1*, nothing occurs 'later', in the illusory future, to real-time cortical consciousness; all events are earlier. All sensory events have a latency because it takes time to access cortical consciousness from the periphery, it also takes time for cortical consciousness to access earlier events in transitory locations that are working or iconic memory. The sensation of time or memory is in reference to this "0" conscious time, and thus reversible in cycling to and from the delayed conscious sensation. While the objective, unidirectional arrow of time is a conscious way to make causal sense of physical reality, internally the brain creates a logic of time by circularly accessing spatial locations in the hippocampus and the cortex, rather than addressing memory of an image literally as stored bits of binary data.

The manipulation of the direction of time necessary for cortex to be in control, is accompanied by an inversion of the plane of the visual field, resulting in a reversed and upside-down retinotopic representation of the visual field in V1 cortex; similarly, a left-right reversal of the dermatomes on the skin's surface occurs at the decussation in the medial lemniscus of the brain stem (that inputs into the VPL), resulting in a representation of the left side of the body on the right side of the somatosensory cortex and vice versa.[92] For cortical tissue to think it is in real time, "0" time has to be at the cortical location. However, the sensory periphery has to be at "0" time, because the receptor is objectively at the emitted time of afferent stimulation. So the brain solves this matching problem by making "Left" facing the brain at proximal sensory input, cross-over to meet "Left" of cortical tissue that receives sensory stimulation. The view from the brain faces 180 degrees to the outer world so that the physical space at its sensory periphery matches symmetrically with the neural space required for conscious sensation and control. That a majority of neurons are corticofugally directed from V1 cortex to the LGN,[93] is a strong indication that V1 cortex is the actual visual organ and not the rapidly trembling eyeballs, and supports the circularly reversible sequencing of time diagrammed in *Fig. 2.1*, in which conscious time initiates in cortex.

The last chapter showed that in the altered virtual position of the image plane from the retina, the z-spike does not discriminate the distance of V1 cortex from that of the retina. Spikes that do not contain or transmit bits of information from components of external space, but rather move the z-locations centered on RGCs, require that the orthogonal percep-

---

[92] Any anatomy text, such as Functional Neuroanatomy by N.B. Everett, shows the sensory decussation at the medial lemniscus, and the corresponding pyramidal decussation for the motor system.

[93] Sherman, S.M. and Guillery, R.W. (2002) Phil. Trans. Roy. Soc. Lond. B 357:1695; Budd, J. (2004) Visual Neurosci. 21:487.

tion of the dimensions of oriented length at V1, at each x-y location, be inverted via corticofugal output back to LGN. While z-spikes primitively react to stimuli without coding, they incrementally converge into anatomical structures that create perceptions required to affect their own input. The transfer of location from the retina, via spikes with no code of z magnitude and no x-y information, requires that the orthogonal plane, the 2D x-y dimension reified in the convergent and divergent circuitry that constitutes the expanded surface area of V1 cortex, has a massive corticofugal effect on LGN input z spikes, a directional disequilibrium imposed by anatomical x-y dimensions converged in V1 oriented simple cell RFs.[94] Corticofugal output to LGN is via thinner and thus slower conducting fibers than is input to V1, so does not communicate information rapidly but may be necessary for synchrony of spikes between LGN and V1. Causality requires V1 to act backward to keep orthogonal maps in the LGN dynamically aligned; corticofugal constraints from elementary V1 perceptions are necessary for timing and locational accuracy of input z spikes.

To summarize, it is possible to make consistent the temporal latency measured at cortex in response to peripheral stimulation and the subjective feeling that the cortex is acting in real time with no conscious sensation of that latency. If different times are rep-

---

[94] Besides locally integrating neurons and neurons that integrate with long horizontal processes, V1 layer 6 neurons relay outputs from superficial layers 2 and 3 that have orientation or 'length-tuned' RFs that organize the concentric RF boundaries of LGN neurons in rows; see McCart, R.J. & Henry, G.H. (1994) Brain Res. 653:351; Gilbert, C.D. (1983) Ann. Rev. Neurosci. 6:217; and Thomson, A.M. (2010) Front. Neuroanat. 4:13. The last author also makes the point that the sustained output of cortico-thalamic cells is not in accord with conventionally defined feedback loop dynamics, a topic to be explored in the next chapter.

resented as sequential anatomical loci, then no illusory referral backward in time is required to explain the Libet experiments, or by consciousness to account for delays in sensation or motor activation. One can have a sense of objective free will at the cortex at "0" time, and not be under the robotic control of prior neural events. However, reflexes occur subliminally; and in persistent disease states, neural substructures do affect emergent conscious events. To the conscious cortex, historical time, or memory, is accessed via a spatial location in cortical layers, distinct from the continuously moving z spike-locations that sense in "0" or real time, with no sense of accumulated time, therefore called the stream of consciousness.

CONCLUSIONS

1) Consciousness is distinguished from memory because it is always in the present. Conscious time has to be the initiating time, and any sense of time, or memory, progresses into the past, backward, from this "0" time. An envisioned, predictable 'future' is also based on extended present realities.

2) The perception of the arrow of time, with which we make cognitive sense of progress and development, is reversed so that one consciously senses that one's decisions are in control, rather than delayed in response to external events.

3) The access of a memory or a time in the past, is a sequential movement of spikes to a neural location, to reestablish a transient past memory consciously at that location. That a time in the past can

be a neural location is facilitated by the insensitivity of single neurons to imposed cognitive definitions of distance and time, which are not reductively 'understood' by a neuron.

4) While visual neurons move the location of retinal imagery to cortex in a temporal sequence, orthogonal perceptions of oriented length in V1 resulting from these aggregated inputs require a massive corticofugal feedback upon the LGN, in an egocentric reversal of time and space, required for perception in the cortex to be in control.

Sustained Firing, Continued

In this chapter, we explore the implications of spikes that move through repeated 2D map arrays. Let us start by examining the meaning of two experiments mentioned earlier. A short stimulus of say, 2 msec, creates a long period of maintained discharge from cat On RGCs of approximately 60 msec. Expanding the stimulus time up to 32 msec duration did not result in a longer period of RGC firing.[95]

How do Off RGCs responding to the same stimulus, affect V1 cortical responses? By using a voltage-sensitive dye with a very short reaction time, investigators found that in ferrets, Off neurons in V1 layer IV delayed firing when a 2 msec light stimulation was turned off, and similarly to RGC's in the above experiment, sustained On V1 response to short light duration was not inhibited.[96] As light duration increased, the rapidity and amplitude of the sustained

---

[95] Levick & Zacks, op. cit., and Levick, op. cit., from Chap. One.

[96] Eriksson, D., Tompa, T., Roland, P.E. (2008) PLoS One 3:e2673.

Off response increased, up to a light duration of 133 msec. For light durations longer than 133 msec, the delay between V1 peak spike On response and V1 peak spike Off response kept a similar 133 msec duration. At light offset, the V1 Off response lasted about 100 msec longer than the terminated V1 On response.

If one can show that cat, ferret, and human neuronal activation dynamics are temporally similar,[97] the duration of AP On response that outlasts the Off response, about 133 msec above, corresponds with the approximate perceptual moment measured in humans.[98] This moment is a measure of the time, from stimulus onset, needed for V1 neurons to integrate sensory inputs as perceived consciously. The greater delay for the Off response, at short stimulus durations, allows time for short On durations to be perceived, but the delay in Off inhibition of long V1 On sustained responses means that a sensory duration of any length gives a V1 On response sustained to be as long as the perceptual moment.

How do sustained APs apply to the masking illusion termed metacontrast? This sensation requires two stimuli, a target (typically, a solid circle or vertical bar) and a mask (a surrounding ring or pair of bars) successively presented to the foveal area, with an asynchrony about half the perceptual moment's duration. Selected here is one of many metacontrast

---

[97] Eytan et al. and Buzsaki et al., op. cit. Chap. One; neural assemblies are nearly scale-free, requiring about 100-200 msec to activate small and large brains. The perceptual moment doesn't increase duration in larger brains, rather spike conduction speeds increase to compensate for increased neural areas needed for perceptual activity.

[98] Efron, R. (1970) Neuropsychologia 8:37; stimulus durations shorter than 120 msec always gave a minimum perceptual moment of about 120 msec; stimulus intensity and area affect the moment's duration.

studies; this one examines spike responses in V1-V2 cortex to mask or target order, asynchronies and durations.[99] These experimenters show forward masking is best if the mask is presented and turned off about 20 msec before target onset, thereby masking initial target visualization. Target spikes in V1-V2 and the target percept are inhibited, the investigators say, by long-lasting excitatory and inhibitory transients induced by turning off the mask. This inhibition of V1-V2 firing prevents the target's spikes from sustaining for the duration needed to be perceived in more distal cortical areas.

In the same group of experiments, a backward mask presented after the target stimulus, inhibits V1-V2 response to the target and its perception. Another study shows that a 16 msec target causes a continued response of 300 msec in cortex; immediately following the target with a mask for 20 msec terminates late cortical target response and perception in 30 msec.[100] The interpretation here, for backward masking in general, is that newly generated RGC mask spikes append to identical, cortical z spikes that have latently summated target timing. The percept in cortical areas distal to V1 shifts to the new retinal mask, even though older, perceptually delayed spikes were initiated by the target.

These findings are logical if z spikes contain no encoded image information. Long-latency spikes in a posterior area of cortex, with no identifying target data, at the same time a spike stimulated by a mask

---

[99] Macknik, S. & Livingstone, M. (1998) Nature Neurosci. 1:144; Macknik, S. & Haglund, M. (1999) PNAS (USA) 96:15208; Macknik, S., Martinez-Conde, S., Haglund, M. (2000) PNAS (USA) 97:7556.

[100] Rolls, E. & Tovee, M (1994) Proc. Biol. Sci. 257:9; IT spike termination correlated with a just noticeable perception of the target.

initiates at the retina, rapidly change perception from the former target to the just-initiated retinal mask. New z spikes add sequentially to older z spikes, so that new imagery is perceived with retinal timing and spatial precision. The new retinal spikes entrain onto previously summated cortical spikes.

Other neurophysiological studies of backward masking have examined the locations of cortical spiking activity that correlate with the perception that the second presented image masks the visibility of the prior target.[101] In two studies with different target and mask durations, investigators found that average and peak spike responses with latencies of 110-121 msec due to the target, were not yet perceived; reentrant posterior cortical spikes from the second masking stimulus, at 160 msec, were thought to overtake and inhibit the earlier activity of the target in distal occipital cortex, to mask target perception.

However, the assumption that spikes encode target information makes paradoxical demands on the cortical processing machinery. The state it is the delayed, perceptual reentrant spikes at 110-121 msec that still contain target information, which are disrupted by the later mask information at 160 msec. Rather than this time-reversed causality based on spike encoding, it is simpler here to say that immediate spikes from the mask at the retina append to the prior identical target-stimulated cortical spikes.

Also, in order to make the inference that reentrant spikes are necessary to make the first target stimulus perceptually invisible, the investigators use average and peak spike responses, which statistically in-

---

[101] Fahrenfort, J., Scholte, J., Lamme, V. (2007) J. Cogn. Neurosci. 19:1488 and (2008) J. Vis. 8:No. 12.

crease response latencies to stimulus onset. Their methods do not separate out the mix of recurrent feedback delays at a recording location; here, initial spike latency to stimulus onset is more relevant, due to the rapid effect of high-contrast retinal mask stimulation to induce a shift in percept. The paradigm here, in which new mask spikes append to identical, prior z spikes that are now latent in posterior cortex, does not require that a mask must have faster reentrant spike looping to inhibit target visibility. Less convoluted is that new retinal spikes perceptually synchronize with identical, now cortical z spikes. Here, z spikes do not transmit encoded mask information, but synchronize older identical z spikes in all areas, with a perceptual latency of about 150 msec, with new retinal mask spikes.[102]

In other experiments, the fastest one or two spikes recorded in a 12.5 msec window 120-150 msec after stimulus onset, correlate with the highest categorization or identification accuracy of a stimulus, measured in primate inferotemporal (IT) cortex.[103] Here, RGC spikes sustain during a fixation that lasts a duration of 150 msec,[104] for perceptual precision. However, a constraint for spikes originating from a region, and synchronized in time at a distant location, is that they cannot move information simultaneously. For spikes to fire in the same phase at two recorded locations, the wavelength period extends

---

[102] Roland, P. (2010) Front. Syst. Neurosci. 4:28.

[103] Hung, C., Kreiman, G., Poggio, T., DiCarlo, J. (2005) Science 310:863; about 8 synapses delay spikes in transit to IT cortex. Sugase, Y., Yamane, S. Ueno, S., Kawano, S. (1999) Nature 400:869, show peak IT spike rates at ~110-150 msec that are sustained over a longer period, perhaps due to a 350 msec stimulus presentation time, compared to the 100 msec stimulation time in Hung et al.

[104] Jung, R. (1973) Handbook of Sensory Physiology 7:3A, p. 87.

to synchronize spike rate with increased neural length. Implicit of a phase-locked frequency is that it is tuned for spike velocities,[105] sustained spike rates and distances from other recorded locations, which in turn depend on the number of synaptic clefts traversed, axon diameters and myelination.[106]

The thinnest, slowest conducting parvocellular neurons[107] from the fovea, also sustain high rates of APs to nearby synapses. Spikes at about 2 meters/sec,[108] sustained at a rate of 100 spikes/sec, should be transiently and repeatedly synchronous at several synaptic junctions in the serial visual arrays of primates.[109] Adjacent RGCs at the retina transmit spikes at the same time,[110] causing synchronized fir-

---

[105] Murakoshi, T., Guo, J., Ichinose, T. (1993) Neurosci. Lett. 163:211, find velocities of .15-.55 m/sec in unmyelinated gray cortical matter; higher speeds of 3.3 m/sec are in corpus callosum (Salami, M., Itain, C., Tsumoto, T., Kimura, F. (2003) PNAS(USA) 100:6174). Excluding synapses, axonal conduction speeds range between 4-20 m/sec (in Innocenti, G., Vercelli, A., Caminiti, R. (2014) Cereb. Cortex 24:2178); a single cortical area has axons of varied diameters and spike velocities originating and terminating in it.

[106] Lachaux, J.-P., Jerbi, K., Bertrand, O., Minotti, L., Hoffmann, D., Schoendorff, B, Kahane, P. (2007) PLoS One, 2:e1094; this reference gives a non-trivial discussion on the correlation of higher electroencephalogram (EEG) frequencies with shorter cortical distances.

[107] We temporarily ignore koniocellular neurons, which conduct slowest from retinal small bistratified cells to the interlaminar layers of the LGN, and stimulate conscious wakefulness in low-light conditions.

[108] Gouras, op. cit., Chap. One; this conduction speed is from primate fovea. Conduction speeds from perifoveal retina are slightly higher in cats, see Stone, J. & Fukuda, Y. (1974) J. Neurophys. 37:722.

[109] Keopsell, K., Wang, X., Vaingankar, V., Rathbun, D., Usrey, W., Hirsch, J., Sommer, F. (2009) Front. Syst. Neurosci. Epub. 3:4; they show phase-locking at retina and thalamus if a sustained rate code is dejittered by synchronizing phase with stimulus timing.

[110] Mastronarde, D. (1989) Trends Neurosci. 12:75; Schnitzer, M. & Meister, M. (2003) Neuron 37:499; Usrey, W. & Reid, R.C. (1999) Ann. Rev. Physiol. 61:435.

ing in the LGN[111] with a 1 msec precision,[112] which is also the approximate delay in a synaptic cleft and the duration of a typical spike.[113] Fixational tremor synchronizes the firing in the layer of RGCs, so that the z spikes marking image edges move with synchronous precision in parallel fibers.[114] Synchronized movement of spikes marks location of the image in parallel neurons of the same P label (with similar axonal spike velocities); this is necessary for a short window of temporal summation at synapses, to reemit spikes to the next level of the visual system. However, z spike synchrony is not required to code image information; if sustained spikes are a temporal code during perception, image x-y data is coded over time, not z-synchronized as here.

Here we must examine what 'synchronous time' means. Conventional information transfer requires a sequential AP stream, with some form of encoding and decoding process, between two spatial locations. But as stated here, a spike is a moving z location, defined in serial arrays by the same x-y coordinates. A high rate of APs creates, at the same objectively measured instant in time, several spikes on the z axis. As discussed already, axonal distance

---

[111] Usrey, op. cit. from Ch. One.

[112] Reinagel, P. & Reid, R.C. (2000) J. Neurosci. 20:5392; Butts, D., Weng, C., Jin, J., Yeh, C., Lesica, N., Alonso, J., Stanley, G. (2007) Nature 449:92; the latter reference states that higher spike precision increases information without bound, even beyond the information in the image itself.

[113] Shu, Y., Yu, Y., Yang, J., McCormick, D, (2007) PNAS (USA) 104:11453; Murakoshi et al., op. cit. Temporal summation and phase-locking may be facilitated by a timely pause at the synaptic cleft.

[114] Greschner et al. op. cit. Ch. One; retinal tremor in turtles, synchronizes RGC spikes in the retinal surface; shown also, is that irregularity introduced into the precision of synchronous RGC spikes can degrade image features.

is not a property sensed by z spikes that have no x-y tag, and orthogonal 2D surfaces repeat independently rather than add into a 3D property. Proximal and distal spikes at repeated x-y loci at the same objective time, are z equivalent. Sustained APs that synchronize, are temporally equivalent z locations in axons through these repeated 2D surfaces, in which enduring, convergent z spikes reemit due to synchronizing x-y tremor. Synchronized temporal equivalence of spikes moving on the z axis, is due to the prior anatomical development and maturation of serial, identically mapped x-y surfaces.

How does this analysis apply to the smooth pursuit of the eyes in following a target's motion (*Fig. 3.1*)? After a momentary lag of about 100 msec following initial movement, a target of constant speed and predictable trajectory is tracked by the fovea seemingly in real time, without oscillating to a final

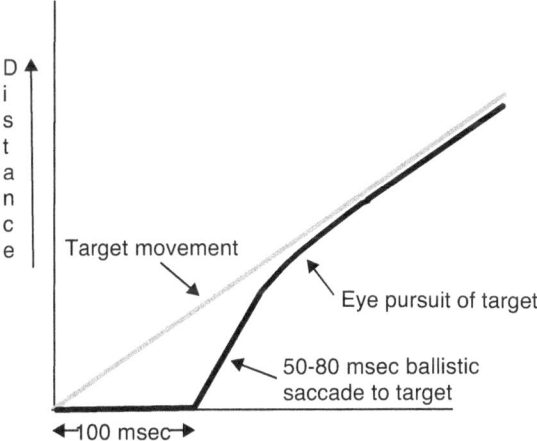

Fig. 3.1: When the visual target moves at constant speed starting at the corner of the graph, it takes almost 100 msec for neural mechanisms to react to this sudden movement, resulting in the foveal saccade to the moving target. After converging onto and smoothly pursuing the target, the moving fovea is able to keep the target centered without lag (drawing adapted from data in first two references on the next page).

position, and without a timing delay in tracking the target.[115] The initial delay in following the changing position of the target is due to the abrupt misalignment of x-y positions of the target and of the fovea. Once new x-y positions of the target on the fovea reestablish a sustained sequence of spikes from the new target location to intervening maps and cortex, we sense that our fovea is precisely on the target as it moves, without temporal lag, hysteresis, or perceived inaccuracy, as would be the case if looping spike information were correcting for the error.[116]

There is no accumulation of error that is periodically corrected, as would be the case with the delay of feedback from the target. The subjective perception that the fovea is directly on the target, corresponds with the objective movement of the target's position, even for periodic motions of various kinds lasting periods of 15 minutes.[117] The ability to track periodic motion over long periods of time without error has traditionally required predictors, both in elec-

---

[115] Rashbass, C. (1961) J. of Physiol. 159:326; Lisberger, G. & Westbrook, L. (1985) J. of Neurosci. 5:1662. Target acquisition by the eyes in converging pursuit (after initial 100 msec delay to respond to target movement) is thought to be a pre-programmed (or ballistic) saccade without feedback, after which slower 'closed-loop' feedback tracks the target. Experimental 'open-loop' conditions disconnect this hypothesized delayed looping feedback, so that the fovea's accurate orientation to target position is annulled.

[116] Shibata, T., Tabata, H., Schaal, S., Kawato, M. (2005) Neural Networks 18:213; an empirical 125 msec response delay follows an abrupt change in smooth target motion; simulated control models of positive feedforward and negative feedback during smooth pursuit of a sinusoidal target, also have the same order of delay, causing pursuit to continually lag the target.

[117] Bahill, A. & McDonald, J. (1983) Vision Res. 23:1573, show graphs of small shifts in foveal position as the fovea pursues a periodic moving target over many minutes, which are errors of eye position, similar to FEMs, that are too quick for cortical feedback, but cause no perception that the target is shifting off the fovea.

tronic feedback and in neurophysiology, but these have delay and concomitant error accumulation also.[118] Here, target motion stimulates a high rate of sustained firing, increasing the temporal coincidence of spikes that transiently synchronize retinal RGCs with distant cortical locations. This synchrony associates the same x-y loci in repeated 2D maps via identical z spikes more quickly than conventional negative feedback, which would require significant delays for spikes to transfer and decode target information between sender and receiver.

Restating this hypothesis, sustained APs from the retina input into succeeding orthogonal maps at the same x-y locations, to create a synchronized firing at near and far maps. The initial delay to pursue a target's abrupt motion suggests that phase-locking, rather than feedback looping, needs time to establish on multiple maps from retina to cortical areas.

When a person detects a target of interest, it takes 100 msec or more for the neural circuitry to bootstrap itself before motor neurons saccade, or switch gaze, to the new target. The saccade, 50-80 msec for the short distance diagrammed in *Fig. 3.1*, is ballistic, that is, rapid but imprecise due to the abruptness of target appearance, so requires a small corrective saccade at termination that lasts a few more msec. However, target location can be corrected even faster than this. If a target is changed to a nearby position while the eyes are saccading to the target of interest, the targeting maps detect this with a very short latency, correcting to the new target after the end of the inaccurate saccade, with

---

[118] Miall, R. & Wolpert, D. (1996) Neural Networks 9:1265 and Miall, R. & Jackson, D. (2006) Exp. Br. Res. 172:77, detail the complications of adding adaptability to, and show evidence against, the Smith predictor and feedforward schemes that require delays for adaptation.

only a few msec increase in total saccade time.[119] Cortical feedback loops could not process information within the minimal 100 msec latency for perception, or during the open-loop ballistic course shown in *Fig. 3.1*, to alter a saccade's final retinotopic position.[120] However, in-process errors can quickly be corrected in local circuitry without cortical feedback, abetted by the short spatial and temporal intervals between sustained z spikes impinging on an orthogonal x-y surface like the SC.

One must also consider that in the last experiment, the presence of already sustained spikes from the initial target shortens the response to the intermediate target. 'Feedback' requires a delay by command centers to spike-encode the information about the changed target. But a shift in target-generated spikes at retinotopic maps, quickly append to already present spikes in higher centers, which here, do not have specific information about targets. If the target moves locally on the SC retinotopic map, this quickens incremental directional firing so that the fovea continuously pursues the slight shift of x-y location.[121] This foveally directed microsaccade is

---

[119] In Goodale, M., Pelisson, D., Prablanc, C. (1986) Nature 320:748. Keller, E., Gandhi, N., Shieh, J. (1996) Vis. Neurosci. 13:1059, alternatively find that a target extinguished before the saccade, and stimulated interruption of the saccade during the saccade, do not stop the saccade from achieving its final target position. This supports the hypothesis here that sustained spikes do not pre-program a target destination, but target-generated spikes continuously change x-y location on the retinotopic map.

[120] Sparks, D. (2002) Nature Reviews Neuroscience 3:952, states that no feedback or error comparator circuits have been found in higher mammals to adjust for amplitude during a saccade.

[121] Krauzlis, R., Basso, M., Wurtz, R. (2000) J. Neurophysiol. 84:876, find that SC 'fixation cells' also pursue the moving target over short distances, to quickly correct small mismatches between the target location and the fovea.

initiated by stimulation of perifoveal sensory RFs that map to motor neurons, located low in the vertical modules that make up the retinotopic sensory-motor layers of the SC.[122] RGC neurons bifurcate to SC and LGN, which then converge to layers with the same retinotopy in V1.[123] The registry of overlying sensory and motor neurons in the SC permits a fast, preprogrammed direction and amplitude response, proportional to fovea vs. target misalignment.

To pursue the question explicitly: how do intense RGC APs generated by moving target edges, translate to the sustained motor APs that control accurate saccades? In primates, it is known that movement responsive V5 cortex is involved, sending signals to the cerebellum and to areas of the frontal cortex, one of which is the frontal eye field (FEF), a cognitive eye targeting area with a high rate of sustained firing.[124] The FEF, V5, and SC have retinotopic maps, as do the cerebellum and brainstem. A sustained motor output from shifting convergent inputs does not require looping feedback.[125] Sustained SC

---

[122] Bergeron, A. & Guitton, D. (2000) Nature Neurosci. 3: 932, examine the sensory-motor coordination of eye movements by SC maps. Isa, T. & Sparks, D. (2006) in Microcircuits: The Interface between Neurons and Global Brain Function. Eds: Grillner, S. & Graybiel, A., p.5, review the precise mapping of intralaminar projections in contiguous sensory-motor layers of the SC. Isa, T. & Hall, W. (2009) J. Neurophys. 102:2581, describe the modular SC wiring of narrow and wide field sensory layer RFs to pre-motor and motor cells.

[123] Bridgeman, B., Kirch, M., Sperling, A. (1981) Percept. Psychophys. 29:336, compare motor accuracy of subliminally sensed motion from the SC, with stable visible input from LGN, on sensory perception.

[124] Schall, J. (1991) J. Neurophysiol. 66:559.

[125] Goldman, M. (2009) Neuron: 61:621. Convergent inputs may sustain motor firing to keep eyeballs fixated without feedback delay, but integration of saccade velocity to position requires more complex circuitry. As described here, sustained firing from serially shifting inputs results from spatial convergence, such as in perifoveal RGCs.

motor cell spiking to maintain eyeball position increases away from the medial nasal position[126]; at the most lateral eyeball position the firing maximizes at over 200 spikes/sec.[127] Saccade amplitude and direction are mapped by a gradient of SC deep layer motor burster cells that ballistically move the eyeball, and sustained cells that keep the eyeball positioned. The VOR referenced in Chapter One, which alters spike rates to keep the eyes fixated as the head moves, is not discussed here.

This aggregate firing of neurons, by its volume and intensity or rate (a population code?), controls the number and volume of muscle fibers activated; the rate of stimulation of local motor cells that are simultaneously activated increases, which creates more force, therefore how far the eyeball turns.[128] The most parsimonious explanation is that sustained spiking is not temporally coded information from a stored memory that stabilizes the eyeball at one position. Rather sustained spikes refresh x-y locations at fovea, SC, and other retinotopic areas that per-

---

[126] Major, G., Baker, R., Aksay, E., Mensh, B., Seung, H., Tank, D. (2004) PNAS (USA) $\underline{101}$:7739, show that velocity and AP burst frequency both increase with the saccade length. They use the evolutionarily simpler goldfish, with motor position cells in Area I, corresponding to areas in the reticular formation of cats and monkeys that control horizontal eye movement. Aksay, E., Olasagasti, I., Mensh, B., Baker, R., Goldman, M., Tank, D. (2007) Nature Neuroscience $\underline{10}$:494; and Aksay, E. Baker, R., Seung, H., Tank, D. (2003) J. of Neurosci. $\underline{23}$:10852, find no neural feedback loops that could cause the firing regularity or synchrony in Area I position cells.

[127] This spike rate is evolutionarily conserved in humans and goldfish, see Sparks, op. cit.; so like the theory expounded here, is brain size invariant; see Eytan et al., Buzsaki et al., op. cit. Chap. One.

[128] Davis-Lopez de Carrizosa, M., Morado-Diaz, C., Miller, J., de la Cruz, R., Pastor, A. (2011) J. Neurosci. $\underline{31}$:2271, use the term 'ensemble innervation' to characterize the overlapping phasic and tonic groups of fibers that create the whole muscle force during the saccade and at saccade's end.

ceive and control motor activity, such as V5 cortex and the FEF, to synchronize ordinarily distant retinotopic maps of a target's sensed location with the matching motor map activity that controls eyeball position. As support for this notion, one can fool the percept of fixation by externally causing the fixation position to slip on the retina; this introduces a compensating change in rate of the motor spike rate that controls eyeball position to maintain target fixation.[129] A simple explanation is that target-stimulated RGC spikes map retinotopically to the SC neurons overlying motor neurons; due to the mismatch of target and fovea, 'fixation cell' spikes emit at a rate and direction to refoveate the target, as in *Fig. 3.2*. In other words, RGC APs abruptly increase as target edges shift off the fovea to a perifoveal SC location; this map error stimulates contiguous motor neurons to fire at high rates, redirecting the fovea to the target at its new external position.

Similarly, if the spike rate that controls the saccadic time course is artificially decreased, motor spikes at retinotopic maps fire for a longer time so that the slow saccade still ends at the final target position.[130] These findings require a convergent mapping between long-latency perception of the target and short-latency subliminal SC motor reactivity to the

---

[129] Major, G., Baker, R., Aksay, E., Seung, H., Tank, D. (2004) PNAS (USA) 101:7745

[130] Soetedjo, R., Kaneko, C, Fuchs, A. (2002) J. Neurophysiol. 87:679, find that sensory feedback does not correct a motor error, but sustains the firing of saccade-related burster neurons for the duration of an artificially slowed saccade to its completion. This is in accord with the hypothesis here, that sustained firing synchronizes multiple retinotopic sensory-motor locations, resulting in an adjustment for the perceived target position on the retina without a calculation of target position temporally coded in feedback, until the mismatch is resolved when the organism cognitively realizes, through phase-locked perception of a match, that the target is on the fovea.

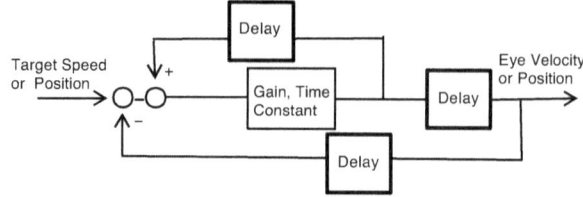

Fig. 3.2a:

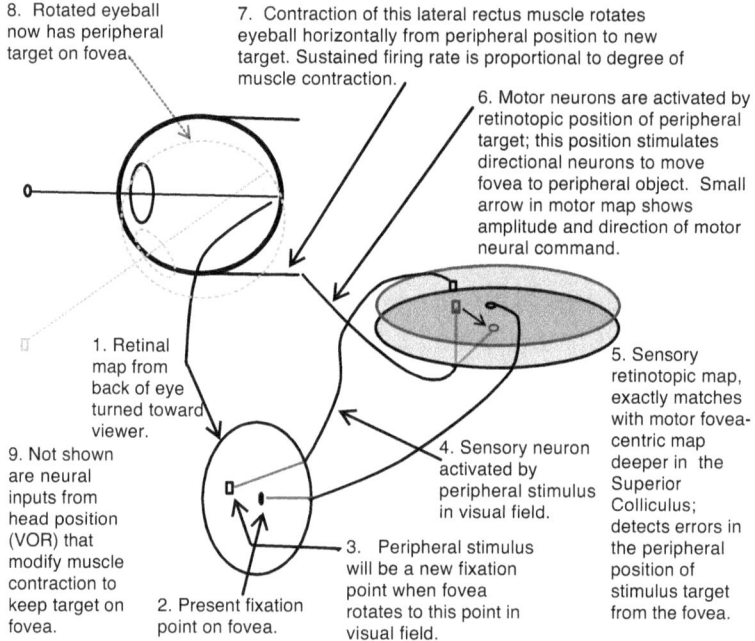

Fig. 3.2b:

Fig. 3.2a: At top is a typical feedback control model for eye movements, with delays due to long loops and branch decision points. 3.2b: The bottom diagram simplifies the redundant maps, but clearly shows that contiguous sensory-motor maps detect small mismatches quickly, and also control larger saccades as shown in sequence 6-8. The whole sequence shows the remapping of the image location so that the current fixation target is always centered on the retinotopic map. A new peripheral target stimulates a motor command to the foveal center of the SC map; the new target's sensory location maps directly to motor neurons that control direction and amplitude. Motor firing rate contracts muscle so the fovea is centered at the formerly peripheral target (drawing from data in Sparks, op.cit., Bergeron et al., op. cit., Sommer et al., op.cit.).

target location. Cortical perception and sensory-motor reactivity coincide via z spikes on repeated retinotopic maps; what is construed as cortical feedback to transmit image information, is actually z spike synchronization at matching x-y locations.

Cortical feedback not only lags speedy SC sensory-motor saccadic responses to visual targets, but is too slow for 2D reaching actions. Altering a target location changes in-progress reaching trajectories with latencies much shorter than reaches lasting several hundred msec.[131] Of importance here is that short reflex loops between the fingers and the cervical spine incorporate proprioception into precise actions, without requiring longer cortical loops to transmit visual targeting information. Vision, and in the blind, proprioception, match perceptual intent with variable, smooth hand trajectories that increase precision closer to the target.[132] Predictive models have been invoked[133] to explain this short latency precision as the arm extends and the hand reaches to a precise grasp of the target. The next chapter shows that phase-locked timing over z distance, at the same repeated x-y location at peripheral, central, sensory and motor maps, can better explain this virtual reduction of neuronal z distance, which increases z timing precision of higher spike rates at successive x-y aligned maps.

---

[131] Dean, H., Hagan, M., Pesaran, B. (2012) Neuron 73:829, Goodale et al., op. cit.; the unseen hand changes course to a new target as soon as a saccade alters course to a new target. Others show visual input latencies that affect in-process reaching to be as short as 100 ms in humans in Pruszinski, J., King, G., Boisse, L., Scott, S., Flanagan, J., Munoz, D. (2010) Eur. J. Neurosci. 32:1049; and 60 ms in cats (Pettersson, L. & Perfiliev, S. (2002) Eur. J. Neurosci. 16:1342).

[132] Gosselin-Kessiby, N., Kalaska, J., Messier, J. (2009) J. Neurosci. 29:3485.

[133] Miall & Wolpert, op. cit.

When the fovea shifts to new targets with large saccades, the visual field also shifts on maps in LGN, SC, V1 and other areas. Is there a need for feedback to remap the transient field shift on the anatomical x-y maps for stability to be perceived? Shifting inputs converge into V1 simple cell RFs that respond to x-y lengths and orientations of image edges. IT cortex, with RFs that cover nearly the whole visual field, responds to object features converged from distributed simple cell RFs, but does not perceive shifting of the object itself. Thus corollary discharge, or efference copy, a motor notice via spikes from the SC to the FEF of impending visual field movement before saccades are initiated, should be construed instead as a synchronization of corresponding x-y points on retinotopic maps.[134] The physical distance between the 2D maps at SC and FEF are constricted by z spikes synchronized at the *same* time, so that these maps are effectively superposed with no z dimension. A new target location overlies the equivalent x-y location on a hard-wired motor map that has the saccadic amplitude and direction to the new target. That this corollary discharge courses from SC via mediodorsal relay thalamus to FEF, almost 100 msec before the actual saccade,[135] allows prior activation of neurons without the delay of post-saccadic perception, at FEF and other cognitively evaluative areas. There is

---

[134] Sherman, op. cit. Chap. One, finds that sensory inputs that map to the LGN always bifurcate to a brainstem motor map.

[135] Sommer, M. & Wurtz, R. (2004) J. Neurophysiol. 91:1381; the initial latency of corollary discharge is 85 msec before the saccade in the SC and diminishes to 54 msec before, in the FEF; the peak of the same spike discharge is 9 msec before in the SC and at 0 msec (= synchrony) before the saccade in the FEF. The latency for corollary discharge in saccades is similar to the lag time for accurate foveation of smooth target motion shown in *Fig. 3.1*, and may serve similarly to synchronize phase-locked activation with intended motor action.

proprioception from the extraocular muscles moving the eyeball, to the somatosensory cortex,[136] but it is too slow to create the perceptual stability of the shifted, newly fixated target; or to compensate, if retinal spikes were encoding the information of the shifting x-y imagery as a convergently integrated sparse code at cortical centers.[137] However, this slow 'feedback' acts over the long term to keep dynamically tensioned maps retinotopically aligned; the small error in ballistic saccades is within the expanded RF areas of cortical maps. If serial maps are aligned, spikes that are temporal z locations, converge within the x-y boundaries that define retinotopic RFs.[138] Here, convergent simple cell RFs distributed in V1 cortex, enable aligned receptors on the 2D retina to detect orientation, despite the lack of x-y coding by RGC z spikes.[139] That microsaccades are not perceived as unstable in V1 cortex,

---

[136] Wang, X., Zhang, M., Cohen, I., Goldberg, M. (2007) Nature Neurosci. 10:640, describe a delayed proprioceptive input to somatosensory cortex that may reach V1 cortex, which they also prove is not a corollary discharge.

[137] Keller, E. & Robinson, D. (1971) J. Neurophysiol. 34:908; Sparks, op. cit., give feedback and feed-forward mechanisms hypothesized to correct for shifts in visual input due to saccades, but no anatomical looping feedback to V1 cortex has ever been found. If z spikes have no image x-y information, a saccadic shift in image location at V1 needs no stabilization.

[138] Sensory image z spikes are transient, while foveal retinotopy is hardwired in SC, LGN, and V1, allowing saccades to targets that are always centered on the fovea. On a longer time scale, reciprocal topographic maps between motor and somatosensory cortex gradually lose alignment, requiring proprioception to calibrate the long-term x-y registry of anatomically aligned maps; in Wang et al, op. cit.

[139] Nakamura, K. & Colby, C. (2002) PNAS (USA) 99:4026 give experimental evidence for low image perception at V1 compared to succeeding visual areas that have a greater perceptual role. Topographical inputs from an image and its perceptions are conmingled in the same cortical areas, but are separable; in Dulin, D, Hatwell, Y., Pylyshyn, Z., Chakron, S. (2008) Neurosci. Biobeh. Rev. 32:1396.

but also are not corrected by imprecise oculomotor control,[140] leaves the synergism developing here: 1) Identical z spikes with no x-y information do not deliver these coordinates onward from proximally shifting RF areas; 2) Edge-generated inputs reemit at slower rates due to increased distance, latency and RF area that accrues at serial 2D synaptic arrays; 3) Serial x-y convergence reemits z spikes, a transform to the unshifting 1D time on each z axis.

The perception of image stability during fixation, means that sustained z spikes created by fixational shifting of midget RGCs keep foveal resolution via least-time z convergence.[141] While a least-time light path in media depends on refractive indices, for a spike the fastest path is the shortest, with the fewest synapses between retina and cortex. However, if shifting cones retain image-specific light information over time, the image shifts also; conventionally, feedback is required to remap the shifting retinal image for V1 sensed stability. But shifting RGC RFs spike transiently at contrasty edges, so light is only seen as straight, rather than bending as cone position shifts. Here, tremor stimulates abrupt z spikes, causing transient x-y alignments of shifting midget RGCs with convergent cortical locations (*Fig. 3.3*). A light focused on a cone causes quick adaptation that reduces spike rate, but sequential stimulation

---

[140] Van Ee, R. & Erkelens, C. (1996) Vis. Res. 36:3827 discuss how the measured inaccuracy of oculomotor feedback cannot compensate for tandem monocular disparities due to head and eye movements, and also cannot explain the precision of stable stereovision and stereo-acuity if tremor and drift are not binocularly coupled.

[141] The shortest route from a receptor to the RGC also is most likely to cause the RGC to fire, shown in Greschner et al., op. cit. Ch. One; also, the shortest path is the major input at the center of the RGC RF, in Bolz, J., Rosner, G., Wassle, H. (1982) J. Physiol. 328:171. Kara & Reid, op. cit. Ch. One, show that the fastest and strongest synaptic connections maintain the precise registry between retinotopic maps.

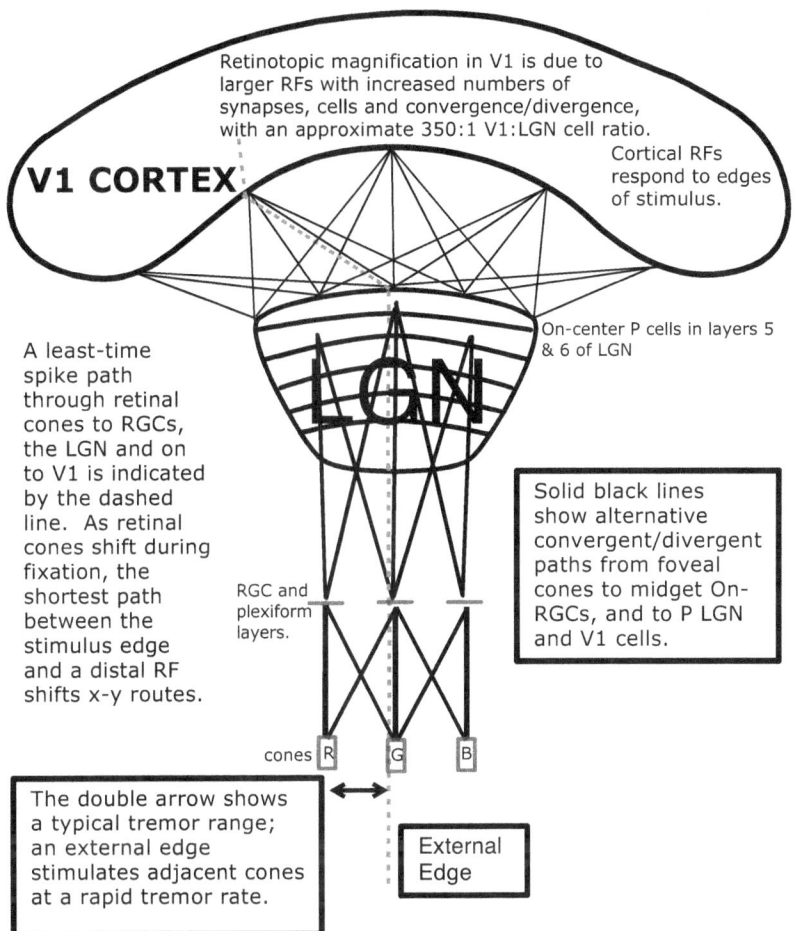

Fig. 3.3: This highly simplified model shows neural divergence and convergence in retinotopically mapped serial arrays. Initial spatial summation from cones occurs at RGCs (Miller, K., Williams, P., Rakic, P. (1990) J. Comp. Neurol. 297:499). RGC and LGN arrays have similar RF areas and cell numbers, which indicates primarily temporal summation. FEMs cross foveal RFs at gamma frequencies, which cause Off and On spikes to alternate from equal numbers of Off and On midget RGCs (Dacey, op. cit. Chap. One). The principle of univariance applies; all cone types in an RGC RF cause it to fire (Li et al. op. cit. Chap. One), but the nearest input to the RF center dominates (Field et al. (2007) op. cit., Chap. One). Rather than a reiterated cortical image that requires stabilizing feedback as it shifts, identical z spikes precisely emitted by abrupt image edges, repetitively align with retinal and V1 RFs at gamma frequencies. The converged, synchronized cortical 1D z spikes do not multiplex 2D data and so do not decode shifting RF data.

of cones that converge to a given LGN cell, sustains LGN spikes;[142] here, RGC x-y shifts align repeatedly, with the z axis of a temporally summating LGN cell.

Other experiments dispute feedback as a source of perceived visual stability. A large background area that moves slowly is perceived to have great stability relative to a small fixated point, which is perceived to move instead.[143] Also, successive fixations integrate in distal RFs, for perception of retinal stability due to longer intervals between z spikes in distal cortex. In addition, the convergence of external space onto the retinal surface, causes a geometric loss of retinal resolution of distant space. If retinal tremor on cortical 2D maps is perceived, distant space jitters with the same amplitude as near space. But the subject sees that spatial resolution is less when fixated on a distant point, so perception in 3D perspective is stable, with no sensed tremor. During fixation, reduced rate cortical z spikes have endured past sustained but subliminal tremor-timed spikes; converging z paths in serial RF-aligned maps, persist as a cortical percept of a stable proximal 2D image.

What else is relevant for the sense of fixational stability? The occurrence of drift and microsaccades diminish with more intense fixation to increase acuity over time.[144] Conventionally, the retinal position

---

[142] Sincich, L., Zhang, Y., Tiruveedhula, P., Horton, J., Roorda, A. (2009) Nature Neurosci. **12**:967; this data supports *Fig. 3.3*.

[143] Bridgeman et al., op. cit.; in the Duncker illusion, the moving image background seems stable because it is larger than the fixation point. This bias may prevent the perception of tremor during fixation, due to the small foveal RF areas relative to the large visual field.

[144] Martinez-Conde, op. cit., Chap. One; Bridgeman, B. & Palca, J. (1980) Vis. Res. **20**:813; moving, not fixed, edges are better stimuli for microsaccades, which suppress during continued fixation requiring high acuity. Microsaccades are also better input to oriented V1 RFs.

of the image would need feedback to stabilize x-y image tremor across receptors, but here, synchronous tremor[145] reemits edge-precise long-latency z spikes so that the fixational percept is spatially stable. Short tremor amplitudes stimulate spikes from the coincidence of image and RF edges of foveal receptors; this dimensional match has highest RGC rates, and thus precision, at contrasty edges. The resulting spike firing pattern is the same whether the retina's fixational movements or external image movements generate them.[146] Fixation upon a stable target therefore does not define absolute coordinates. Because all fixations center on the same neurally wired fovea invariantly located on the SC and other retinotopic maps (*Fig. 3.2*), the previous fixation point is unneeded as a reference; the fovea is self-centered at (0,0) no matter where it fixates.

Accompanying these egocentric foveal fixations, ballistic saccades traverse the SC map's absolute x-y distances from the current fixation point to new targets. During the rapid course of large saccades, shifting of the visual field across V1 is perceptually suppressed, coinciding with transiently reduced spikes.[147] V1 neurons reduce response similarly to

---

[145] Spauschus, A., Marsden, J., Halliday, D., Rosenberg, J., Brown, P, (1999) Exp. Br. Res. 126:556.

[146] Leopold, D. & Logothetis, N. (1998) Exp. Br. Res. 123:341; Snodderly, D., Kagan, I., Gur, M. (2001) Vis. Neurosci. 18:259; Greschner et al., op. cit. Chap. One. The lack of differentiation of self from nonself movement in neurons of visual cortex may explain the jitter aftereffect that is perceived after cortical adaptation to random noise, in the illusion described by Murakami, I. & Cavanagh, P. (1998) Nature 395:798.

[147] Bridgeman, B., Hendry, B., Stark, L. (1975) Vis. Res. 15:719; Wurtz, R.H. (1969) J. Neurophys. 32:975; Burr, D., Morrone, M., Ross, J. (1994) Nature 371:511. The suppressed V1 M response prevents the perception of moving retinal images as the eyes shift from point to point during saccades.

saccadic image shifts and external imagery experimentally moved at the same speed.[148] Therefore feedback to correct absolute internal coordinates cannot govern image stability; but the egocentric perception of stability during fixation is aided by cognition of external references in the FEF area and in the hippocampus (discussed in the next chapter). Here, the subject's percept of an unmoving visual field, despite shifts of imagery across the fovea and V1, requires that light rays at edges are of high contrast,[149] via directionally selective receptors (the Styles-Crawford effect), and concomitant least-time z spikes to perceptual RFs; therefore least-time light rays are an intrinsically stable reference. Emphatic but transient z spikes in RGC, LGN and cortex are not a sparse code, but use edge contrast to synchronize timing,[150] a necessity at synapses to reemit onward spikes. Contrasty edges align retinotopic maps, thereby orienting via an impedance match of rays of photons and neural least-time at the retinal interface. Spikes due to low contrast are few and unreliable, as noise, they do not converge at the

---

[148] Wurtz, R.H. (1969) J. Neurophys. 32:987.

[149] Saccades in dark experimental conditions are increasingly inaccurate, indicating that straight light rays are an important reference necessary to perceive the stability of visual targets; Becker, W. & Klein, H. (1973) Vis. Res. 13:1021.

[150] Sclar, G., Maunsell, J., Lennie, P. (1990) Vis. Res. 30:1; these researchers measure a high spike rate to the same high contrast edge in RFs from RGCs to V5 cortex. Frazor, R. & Geisler, W. (2006) Vis. Res. 46:1585, measure invariant contrast responses in V1 despite changes in many stimulus qualities, including intensity. Neurons respond to the range of light intensity by convergent successive reductions in firing rates to cortex, but respond to contrast independently of intensity, preferentially 'encoding' an invariant contrast response, in van Hateren, J. & Snippe, H. (2006) J. Comp. Physiol A 192:87. As stated here, this exaggerated, invariant response to high contrast edges synchronizes retinal x-y position via spike z-locations (in the M system), and with other RGCs (in the P system) responding to changes in stimulus intensity by scaling changes in spike rate.

next synapse synchronously to emit onward spikes, so do not endure in time to be perceived.[151]

So, why is an afterimage perceived to shift during saccades, even though it stays at the same hard-wired (0,0) foveal position? If a persisting afterimage has been induced, the subject sees the afterimage shift across the visual field during the saccade. Normally, spikes emitted by M RGCs are suppressed in V1 cortex during saccade transit, which assists the perception of stability. But an afterimage, due to saturated rods that keep stimulating RGC spikes, endures due to reemission.[152] Rods and cones input to the same convergent M RGCs in macaques; as spike output saturates,[153] persisting afterimage colors, loss of resolution and shifting are perceived. These saturated rates that imprecisely summate in the large M RFs, also input to V1 simple cells to perceptually dominate P blob inputs,[154] which mediate fixational image resolution and stability.[155] Para-

---

[151] Lesica, N., Jin, J., Weng, C., Yeh, C.-I., Butts, D., Stanley, C., Alonso, J. (2007) Neuron 55:479.

[152] Adelson, E. (1982) Vis. Res. 22:1313.

[153] Cao, R., Lee, B., Sun, H. (2010) J. Vision 10:4, examine rod (responsive to low luminance) and cone (preferring high light intensity) inputs to M RGCs with mesopic light levels that induce afterimages.

[154] Vidyasagar, T., Kulikowski, J., Lipnicki, D., Dreher, B., (2002) Eur. J. Neurosci. 16:945; M and P inputs converge on 25% of V1 cells.

[155] Feedback supposedly explains why stability is disrupted by pressing the edge of the eyelid; the reasoning is that the finger press is not in the normal feedback loop for image stability, so a shifting visual field is sensed. The 2D retina's movement, sensed by M receptors and proprioception, responds to the finger press to create a cortical sense that the visual field is moving during the press. These abnormal 2D inputs dominate the normal timing of retinal inputs to convergent neurons that perceive 3D imagery. Cortical perception, if veridical, has to know an external abnormal source (the finger press) has perturbed image stability. A feedback mechanism should not correct this abnormal disturbance; visual instability should be perceived.

doxically, saturated high spike rates are used as a measure of a neuron's optimal stimulus response.

Convergence and divergence to V1 cortex (see *Fig. 3.3*),[156] creates enlarged RFs with rougher boundaries as seen with current technology, despite the initial strict mapping between RGCs and LGN.[157] The coarse V1 image seen by the external observer is not seen by the subject,[158] who perceives only the synchronized times of z spikes that endure into long-latency perception. Several cones input to LGN P cells, which input to V1 cortical P cells that occupy the centers (called 'blobs') of the pinwheels of oriented simple cells, distributed regularly in V1 cortex, mentioned in Chapter One.[159] The simple cells con-

---

[156] See also *Fig. One* in Kara & Reid, op. cit. Chap. One; also, Peters et al, op. cit. Chap. One, and Peters, A. & Payne, B. (1993) Cereb. Cort. $\underline{3}$:69.

[157] Kara & Reid op. cit. Chap. One, find that 1-3 cat RGCs map to one LGN cell. Sincich, L., Adams, D., Economides, J., Horton, J. (2007) J. Neurosci. $\underline{27}$:2683 explore the response of primate RGC-LGN cells to focused light, with neuro-muscular blockade to eliminate fixational tremor that would expand the number of inputs, and light limited to the center of cone RFs. Midget RGCs show substantial divergence to the LGN. Individual cones stimulated with precisely aimed laser light, that input through midget RGCs to converge on a recorded P LGN cell, show that one cone stimulates the highest LGN spike rate and is also the shortest in neural distance; also Sincich et al. (2009), op. cit.

[158] Nishimoto, S., Vu, A., Naselaris, T., Benjamini, Y., Yu, B., Gallant, J. (2011) Curr. Biol. $\underline{21}$:1641.

[159] Primate V1 cortex perceives acuity because almost half of LGN outputs bypass layer 4C alpha oriented simple cell RFs with horizontal projections, to instead input in 4C beta, with circular non-oriented RFs. The latter P cells vertically project, without horizontal processes, through to V1 layers 2, 3, 5 and 6. In contrast, cat LGN afferents synapse only on oriented V1 cells (cats have few non-oriented cells), without the added primate synapses and projections. Cats, with the many-to-one mapping of receptors to cat foveal RGCs, only have receptor acuity that is not perceptual; see Latawiec et al., op. cit. Chap. One; Livingstone, M. & Hubel, D. (1984) J. Neurosci. $\underline{4}$:309; Blake, R. (1978) Frontiers of Visual Science (Cool, S. & Smith, E., eds.) p. 209.

verge inputs from colinear, adjacent retinal receptors; temporal and spatial summation transiently increase simple cell RF area.[160] Simultaneous or sequential timing of z spikes in long simple cell RFs create feature or motion percepts, respectively. In contrast, P neurons in V1 blobs fire spontaneously, an effect of low threshold sensitivity, similar to the characteristic noisy firing of midget RGCs in the fovea. This is strong evidence that dispersed blob P cells repeat the foveal map for V1 awareness[161] of x-y resolution, due to low P cell spatial integration. The lack of a movement-sense by P cells, supplements in V1 the egocentric foveal (0,0) centering due to retinotopic SC/LGN input, to create awareness of external visual stability. But M inputs into larger spatially and temporally convergent simple cell RFs that surround blob P cells, detect motion past a single receptor, so that a moving large visual background, as described in Bridgeman et al. (1981), quantitatively dominates the inputs to foveal P cells in V1. The egocentric stability perceived as output from RF edge-aligned V1 blob cells, is outcompeted perceptually by the larger spatial convergence of motion inputs in larger V1 M RFs, which may have more survival value for the organism. Experimentation may reveal how external motion-initiated spikes that converge in V1 M RFs, reemitted to larger V5 RFs, dominate the perceived stability temporally summated and reemitted at reduced rate by small V1 foveal P RF edges, which transiently align with image edges during fixation.

---

[160] Kara & Reid, op. cit. Chap. One, show the temporal course of RGC and V1 RF overlap after stimulation; RFs at RGC and V1 increase in diameter with a similar time course up to 23 msec, but the expanded V1 RF lasts longer by 22 msec. As in Lund et al., op. cit. Chap. One, the RF increases due to convergent and divergent inputs over time.

[161] Crick, F. & Koch, C. (1995) Nature 375:121.

This interpretation that long latency RF edge-aligned z spikes at slow rates are perceived cortically, while short latency FEM-generated spikes are too rapid and jitter in x-y location, so are subliminal perceptually, is consistent with experiments that show that visibility of stimuli makes them discriminable, while the same stimuli made subconsciously ambiguous by lowered contrast, increased masking or lessened attention, retain only a probabilistic detectability.[162] Using the concepts here, if the stimulus is less discernible, this reduces the number of z spikes that can rapidly synchronize at synapses to propagate onwards into conscious, long-latency perception.

Paradigms for object identification in IT cortex should consider that the spikes that remain after serial temporal and spatial summations, are only z locations with no labels.[163] Simple cell RFs respond to features of a primate face, sending z spikes to IT neurons[164] without sequentially coding face size, orientation, or location on the V1 map. The many RGC types[165] respond selectively to distinctive external features. Fast-spiking interneurons inhibit slower divergent inputs to favor spikes that due to

---

[162] King J. & Dehaene, S. (2014) Philos. Trans. Roy. Soc. B 369: 20130204.

[163] Hung et al., op. cit., discuss the anomaly that just one or two spikes compute object identity in the initial 12.5 msec of arrival at IT cortical cells. Here, sustained retinal spikes are z-locations in labeled neurons, which synchronize complex retinal information with initial precisely timed, rapidly reemitted convergent IT unlabeled z spikes.

[164] Peretti, D., Rolls, E., Caen, W. (1982) Exp. Br. Res. 47:328; Peretti, D., Smith, P., Potter, O., Mistlin, A., Head, A., Milner, A., Jeeves, M. (1984) Human Neurobiol. 3:197.

[165] Field, G. & Chichilnisky, E. (2007) Ann. Rev. Neurosci. 30:1 and Sanes, J. & Masland, R. (2015) Ann. Rev. Neurosci. 38:221, list 20 to 30 RGC types that detect specific features; Pang, J., Gao, F., Wu, S. (2002) J. Neurosci. 22:4693 describe at least 12 bipolar cell types.

convergent temporal and spatial synchrony, reemit rapidly.[166] Repeated modules of V1 simple cells re-emit into the large RFs of IT cells; a rotating object sustains z spikes, from any x-y locus, that least-time synchronize at an IT location. Ultimately, the data-identical spikes generated by edge-crossings of labeled retinal receptors, synchronize at IT, via the tremor-gated image edge-crossings that stimulate and phase-lock proximal z spikes at distal IT cortex.

Similarly, while in pursuit of a target's motion, the M system at V5 passes z spikes that have no x-y tags but have precise timing, generated by passage of a moving edge, which transiently synchronize V5 with active retinal x-y locations. That sensation and motor maps have contiguous SC x-y locations, are shown in experiments that dissociate subjective perception of smooth target motion from the neuronal motor activity that follows the motion; these both access the same x-y resolution of sensory information. In repeated trials, the 100-150 msec delay by the neuronal mechanisms that sense and initiate the pursuit to the target as it starts moving (*Fig. 3.1*), have a consistent timing variance of 6-10 msec from trial to trial in any individual primate. Though the time of onset of target motion is unknown by the primate beforehand, this behavioral lock of pursuit initiation to the start of target motion is very reliable from trial to trial, in contrast to the more variable behavioral characteristics of pursuit speed and direction as the target starts moving.[167] While neuron

---

[166] Tamas, G., Buhl, E., Somogyi, P. (1997) J. Physiol. 500:715.

[167] Osborne, L., Bialek, W., Lisberger, S. (2004) J. Neurosci. 24:3210; Osborne, L., Lisberger, S., Bialek, W. (2005) Nature 437:412; Osborne, L., Hohl, S., Bialek, W., Lisberger, S. (2007) J. Neurosci. 27:2987. Rasche, C. & Gegenfurtner, K. (2009) Vis. Res. 49:514; early perceptual precision is exceeded by oculomotor precision later.

populations may increase precision by integrating over the time of pursuit, foveal speed and direction in pursuit of the target does not become as precise as perceptual estimates of target speed and direction until after 200-300 msec. In M neurons, only 10 spikes sustain fire in 100 msec. Therefore, the first spike is thought to have the precise timing to initiate smooth pursuit.[168] Here, rather than massive neural computation, a 10 msec precision requires only an orthogonal SC map that rapidly distinguishes target vs. foveal x-y locations via emitted z spikes, which are perceived in 150 msec as distal arrays synchronize with retinotopic maps. Discussion in Chapter Five shows that an added 150 msec sums spikes on all proximo-distal z axes, to synchronize cortical perceptual estimates with retinotopically mapped tracking of the target.

Contiguous sensory-motor maps only partly explain the 10 msec precision of smooth pursuit that starts 100-150 msec after the target starts moving.[169] It takes 45-70 msec after stimulus presentation for spikes to reemit from V1 neurons;[170] later cortical

---

[168] Gollisch, T. (2009) HFSP Journal 3:36, states that latency of the first spike has all the target data; but latency depends on the neuron type (such as OFF or ON), axon diameter and summation speed.

[169] Osborne et al. (2005), (2007), op. cit.; the 10 msec initiating precision results despite very few APs in V5 cortex; neurons on the SC map react quickly to target-foveal discrepancies, in Krauzlis, R. & Dill, N. (2002) Neuron 35:355. A temporal code for target position, direction and speed would be longer than required for SC map matching.

[170] Nowak, L. & Bullier, J. (1997) in Cerebral Cortex, Rockland, K.S., Kaas, J., Peters, A. eds, p. 204; integration time required for each synapse to fire is an unavoidable delay in measuring conduction speed. Reich, D., Mechler, F., Victor, J. (2001) J. Neurophys. 85:1039, show that the shortest visual cortex latencies from receptors in macaques, at 45 msec, are due to maximum edge contrast, which issues the highest rates of RGC spiking to reduce synaptic summation time. Besides contrast, increased stimulus intensity measured as increased luminance and/or retinal area, reduce summation time at synapses.

stages require 100-150 msec. At a frequency of 100 spikes/sec sustained at V1 cortex,[171] equivalent z spikes traverse synaptic stages every 10 msec. An image could not be reconstructed in detail in V1 from information-coding spikes starting at 45 msec of the 150 msec perceptual moment; but identical z spikes that transit every 10 msec to V1 cortex contain a retinally emitted time that is transient at each stage of serial maps to IT cortex. Spikes from initial smooth pursuit of a target sustain, to reemit as long distance/latency spike intervals at large cortical RFs, which perceive retinotopic target deviations. These latent, distal z spikes are synchronous in time with concurrent spikes that modify target and foveal x-y loci every 10 msec at SC, LGN and V1 maps, sustained at gamma rates by jittering retinal receptors.

That synchronous z spikes reduce the apparent distance and time between RF-aligned cortical loci, is shown when sudden image changes cause anticipatory responses in cortex.[172] Neuronal synchrony between motor cortex and the corticospinal column is highest, when the behavioral readiness to respond is greatest, improving motor reaction time by 50 msec.[173] Identical spikes that temporally synchronize, correlate proximal information distally; phase-locked z spikes repetitively fuse topographically aligned surfaces as a single z equivalent site.

---

[171] This rate in both M and P neurons is physiologically realistic, despite lower average cortical spike rates stimulated by light flicker, because high-frequency bursts of spikes generated by microsaccades and stimulus edges traverse synapses with great efficacy; in Macknik & Livingstone, op. cit.; Chichilnisky, E. & Kalmar, R. (2003) J. Neurosci. 23: 6681; also in Martinez-Conde, op. cit. Chap. One.

[172] Roelfsema, P., Engel, A., Konig, P., Singer, W. (1997) Nature 385: 187; visual, parietal and motor cortices rapidly phase-lock in alerting cats.

[173] Schoffelin, J., Oostenveld, R., Fries, P. (2005) Science 308:111.

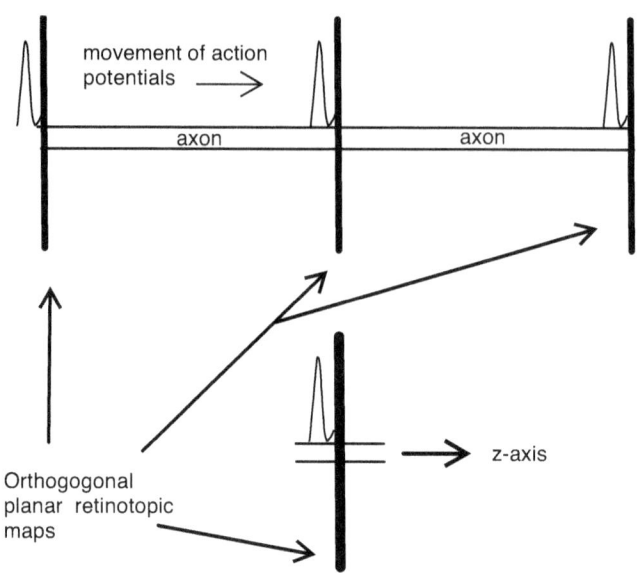

Fig. 3.4: Spikes at the top of the figure are shown as they move in the plane of this page, past multiple retinotopic maps, at the same orthogonal x-y location on each map at the same time. Z distance, emission rates and spike speed synchronize so that spikes phase-lock at each map. A normal viewer of this page has a view equidistant from the repeated 1D z-axis spikes, facilitating the comprehension that they exist simultaneously though sequentially generated in time. With identical spikes phase-locked at 2D surfaces over repeated distances, shown at top, the bottom view reifies the concept that repeated gaps between 2D surfaces do not have temporally cumulative properties when phase-locked. At a sustained frequency of 100 spikes/sec, identical z spikes move with gaps of 10 msec, yet repeatedly persist during 100 msec, to create the illusion that repeated 2D surfaces are a repeatedly transient 2D surface or are dynamic in 3D. This view on a 2D page is a more explicit, orthogonal version of Fig. 2b in the first chapter.

Given that neurons move z spikes between retinotopically mapped x-y locations, can one explicitly test the idea that at synchronized spike frequencies, z locations move, rather than information between stationary x-y-z locations, as experiments based on stimulus-response delay have always suggested? Between RGCs and V1 cells, spikes have a much shorter latency[174] than the 70-100 msec required for maximal cone response after abrupt stimulation of the retina.[175] But the shift of firing from the edge of a midget RGC to another during tremor of nearly 100 Hz, sustains spike firing at initial convergent synapses about every 10 msec, to bridge the delays in receptor and plexiform layer graded potentials that here, are not moving image information. The longer temporal intervals between z spikes in higher order neurons, override the retinal response delays that are subliminal. Rather than transferring coded imagery over time from the retina,[176] it is more efficient in a lengthy neuron for identical z spikes to synchronize their coupled locations/times at transient x-y alignments as retinal receptors shift.

Analog information, such as smear from retinal motion, is not suitably coded by digital spikes with durations of about one msec.[177] The graded potentials

---

[174] Kara & Reid, op. cit. Chap. One; the 5-9 msec latency measured in cats traverses two synapses in about half the neuronal distance and number of synapses measured in primates; it excludes receptor stimulation time, the processing time of slow graded potentials in the horizontal layers of the retinal plexus and divergent slower pathways.

[175] Wang, Y. Weick, M., Demb, J. (2011) J. Neurosci. 31:7670; mouse cones, similar to human foveal cones, have a faster peak response to more intense stimulation; spike rate is generally proportional to cone response. Nikonov, S., Kholodenko, R., Lem, J., Pugh, E. (2006) J. Gen. Physiol. 127:359; a 20 msec stimulus generates a cone response lasting 200 msec. O'Brien, B., Isayama, T. Richardson, R., Berson, D. (2002) J. Physiol. 538.3:787 show millisecond RGC responsiveness that quickly detects motion past a single converging receptor.

[176] deRuyter van Steveninck, R., Laughlin, S. (1996) Nature 379: 642, give evidence that graded potentials have five times the information of the highest spike rates.

[177] One may argue that analog information can be modified if the shape of a spike is broadened by glutamate or other substances that affect ionic currents in the axon membrane. But these effects are very local, and affect spike shape only temporarily. See Sasaki, T., Matsuki, N., Ikegaya, Y. (2011) Science 331:559.

in the plexiform dendritic fields align receptor RFs with RGC types that select image features,[178] rather than slowly processing data. Identical APs from an RGC array define stimulus timing and intensity, but otherwise have little coding of features that enable cortical recognition.[179] Least-time z spikes that re-emit from serial synapses result from x-y synchronized patterns of RGC spikes from connected edges.

The many types of RGCs emit spikes with different shapes and latencies, which affect how quickly spikes are generated, but do not specifically encode stimulus features.[180] However, specific RGC types react to increased stimulus intensity by generically increasing spike rate. For example, rods and blue-sensitive cones converge to the same small bistratified RGC; only rods stimulate spikes at low light levels; as light intensity increases, blue cones gradually stimulate additional spikes from the RGC. A shift to differently shaped spikes with blue information, does

---

[178] Ten plexiform layers, each specific to the dendritic fields of specialized bipolar and RGC types, are described in Pang et al., op. cit.; Sanes & Masland, op. cit, review the many RGC types.

[179] Koch, K., McLean, J., Segev, R., Freed, M., Berry, M., Balasubramanian, V., Sterling, P. (2006) Curr. Biol. $\underline{16}$:1428; spike statistics differ much more between neuron labels than between stimulus features. Berry, M., Warland, D., Meister, M. (1997) PNAS (USA) $\underline{94}$:5411 show that only three features could possibly be temporally coded in a neuron's spike train with an information encoding capacity of 160 distinct time intervals. So spike timing cannot code the complexity of features in a typical object or face.

[180] Different types of RGCs have different spike durations, a measurement which, in turn, is inversely proportional to the differing peak spike rates of each RGC type; in O'Brien et al. op. cit. Stimulus intensity that increases spike rate may decrease spike amplitude, due to limited spike-generation capacity in the neuron; in Meister, M., Pine, J., Baylor, D. (1994) J. Neurosci. Methods $\underline{51}$:95. A steeper spike shape due to the concerted activity of sodium conductance channels increases the speed of spike dynamics, which allows higher spike frequencies to be passed, in Naundorf, B., Wolf, F., Volgushev, M. (2006) Nature $\underline{440}$:1060. Spikes are identical within these limits.

not accompany this increase in spike rate, although increased rate may be construed as more information.[181] Rather the identical spikes have to be transmitting the retinotopic RGC intensity of diffuse light, rather than multiplexing rod and cone x-y defined data. That the small bistratified RGC type is specifically for low-resolution, low-light responsiveness is evident, because only spike rate increases as rod input shifts to blue cone input. The low spike rate at low light levels in this RGC type sustains for a long period; this low spike rate permits the cortex to sense a constant background of low intensity, rather than abrupt changes over time. One may generalize that a higher spike rate corresponding to greater stimulus intensity, traverses convergent synapses with greater efficiency to create stronger and faster perceptions in cortical areas, in this case of diffuse blueness.[182]

Can the response to sequential motion in the same V1 simple cell RF be compared with the response to

---

[181] Crook, J., Davenport, C., Peterson, B., Packer, O., Detwiler, P., Dacey, D. (2009) J. Neurosci. 29:8372; figures show an increasing small bistratified RGC spike rate as the shift from rods to cones occurs at higher light intensity. The rate of identical spikes increases due to faster cone reaction to light level than by rods. Cao et al., op. cit., show that rod and cone inputs to M RGCs combine linearly with increased light intensity, prior to the saturation of output spike rate. Pang, J.-J., Gao, F., Wu, S. (2003) J. Neurosci. 23:2063, also show that increased light intensity causes increased rate and duration of fire of stereotypically identical APs from a mouse alpha-RGC receiving convergent cone and rod input. Additionally, Off and On inputs to the same RGC emit identical spikes, except for a 20 msec offset, in Uchiyama, H., Goto, K., Matsunobu, H. (2001) Neural Netw. 14:611.

[182] Convergence of several blue cones on one RGC mediates diffuse vision, because in the fovea, high resolution requires correspondence of an On cone to one midget RGC. Bipolar cells, at times, emit spikes rather than graded potentials from cone stimulation, so may transmit transient increases in spatial resolution. See Dreosti, E., Esposti, F., Baden, T., Lagarado, L. (2011) Nature Neurosci. 14:951; Saszik, S. & DeVries, S. (2012) J. Neurosci. 32:297.

simultaneous spike inputs on the same cells,[183] corresponding to a stimulus feature (synchronized by RGC outputs?)[184] Dendritic fields and axonal arborizations seem designed for graded potentials; how does the complex integration of labeled neurons in perceptual cortex affect what is sensed at peripheral receptors, or vice versa? Can the long latency of z spikes at IT cortex be perceptually distinguished from fixationally sustained, x-y aligned retinal spikes? Another time question: since the average frequency of APs in IT cortex increases upon object stimulation, and the initial one or two spikes categorize and identify it,[185] is it necessary that late IT spikes synchronize with the retinal spikes that still issue with fixation on the object? Finally, is the perceptual moment solely in z spikes moving in axons to IT cortex, or also in diffuse orthogonal potentials?

Motor coordination is required for a batter to hit a professionally pitched baseball; similarly to foveal initiation of target pursuit, hitting the ball requires a perceptual-motor coordination of less than ten milliseconds.[186] This accuracy is faster than a code

---

[183] M and P neurons input on the same convergent oriented V1 cells (Lund et al. op. cit. Chap. One). Also relevant to M and P cell specificity is that inhibitory feedback on the dendrites or soma of V1 cells determines whether a contrast invariant signal is passed with little orientation selectivity, or is scaled to a reduced response magnitude with sharpened orientation selectivity, in Ma, W., Lu, B., Li, Y., Huang, Z., Zhang, L., Tao, H. (2010) J. Neurosci. 30:14371.

[184] RGCs synchronize output, in Greschner et al. op. cit. Chap. One.

[185] Hung et al., op. cit.; most data here is from primate IT; the human anatomical equivalent is subdivided into areas with different terminology, but we use 'IT' for nominal consistency and simplicity.

[186] Land, M. & McLeod, P. (2000) Nature Neurosci. 3:1340. With repetition of an edge across a receptor's RF, a spike initiates at the same point in its RF (Greschner et al., op. cit. Chap. One). So convergent timing at binocular neurons can have temporal (therefore spatial) acuity finer than the minimal 10 msec spike interval.

of information transmitted from retina to cortex, so requires, if not predictors, then the sustained continuity of synchronized z locations from retina to cortical levels, to coordinate perception with sensory-motor precision. The perceptual moment that integrates a fixated scene is about 4 times longer than the 33 msec required at a typical film frame rate to temporally fuse frames together.[187] If LGN anatomy mediates the temporal continuity of retinotopically matching film images, then the neuronal delay to abrupt external movement via the fast M neurons to perceptual V5 cortex, about 80 msec, must occur without delaying the continuous perceived stimulus position by 80 msec.[188] Here, convergent, large RF V5 synapses that reemit fewer spikes do not require a cortical predictive mechanism to perceive motion as if in real time; rather previously emitted, identical V5 spikes synchronize with newly emitted spikes in serially aligned M RGC RFs as they respond to incremental motion.[189]

This discussion requires an explanation of the flash-lag phenomenon. For this version of the experiment, identical flashes are created at the same time in adjacent moving and stationary stimuli aligned on

---

[187] Butts et al. (2007), op. cit., examine how spike precision affects perceived resolution of film that has fixed frame intervals; they aver that precise spike times at each frame are physiologically unrealistic. Here it is stated that frames fuse due to temporal summation of imprecisely timed spikes. The exact overlap of frames in x-y mapped layers of LGN, has no image degradation because the temporal jitter of z spikes has no x-y information. The retinal x-y map remains in retinotopic register in the first maps of the visual pathway.

[188] Eagleman, D. & Sejnowski, T. (2007) J. Vis. $\underline{7}$:3; the hypothesis is that 'motion bias' shifts the predicted position of a target forward due to a 'postdictive' delay in neural processing of the moving target.

[189] Westheimer, G. & McKee, S. (1977) Vis. Res. $\underline{17}$:887; they estimate that this rapid percept must be sourced in the retina, but do not give a mechanism.

a screen. One might expect that the simultaneous flashes would be perceived in spatial proximity; instead the moving stimulus flash is perceived to be advanced, as if its position is predicted. Intrinsic to the explanation here is that a simple cell has both M and P inputs,[190] corresponding respectively, to sequential motion detection and stationary feature detection, as discussed earlier. But because the moving and the stationary flash stimulate the same convergent simple cells, perceiving cortical neurons confound identical spikes from the same retinal location. P and M retinal receptors discriminate responses to stationary and moving stimuli; but with perceptual delay, merge timing of identical spikes (without divergent M or P data) at convergent cortical cells. Cortical perceptual lag to the abrupt stationary P RGC response synchronizes with a matching delayed, therefore moved, retinal M RGC RF location of the M spikes just stimulated by movement.

Can rapid motion perception be accounted for, with a mechanism that also explains the empirical precision in hitting a baseball? A pitched ball sustains RGC spikes; by aligning with earlier cortical spikes from the same ball, the approaching ball may be perceived more quickly. Abruptly stimulated spikes that converge within a short temporal window maximize spike rate in binocular V1 cells, which also correlates with maximal psychometric perception of 3D distance.[191] New RGC-generated spikes syn-

---

[190] Lund et al., op. cit., Chap. One.

[191] Read & Cumming, op. cit. Chap. One; Trotter, Y. (1995) Perception 24:267; Poggio, G., Gonzales, F., Krause, F. (1988) J. Neurosci. 8:4531. Primate V1 cells with interocular delays with a mean of about 4 msec (the difference in latency to the same V1 cell from the left and right eyes), tolerated a difference of 15-20 msec latency for maximal spike rate. Cells in V1 layers that increase rate at one vergence angle are mixed with cells responsive to other vergence angles.

chronize with spikes generated earlier, in cortically aware areas, as a fastball rapidly closes on the batter. However, motor and perceptual delays that would result from retrieving stored information of the ball's direction as it changes, mean that RGC spikes input to subliminal short-latency areas such as the SC.[192] Here, rather than long processing to predict a ball path, SC layers rapidly register x-y changes in the looming position of the ball. Larger, more rapid changes in the position of a curve ball or slider, emit spikes with less accuracy due to x-y misaligned foveal RGC and V1 RFs. That new RGC spikes append to identical z spikes generated earlier but perceptually older in cortical RFs, can explain how cortical perception synchronizes with the RF aligned fastball. So initially, a distant baseball establishes a delayed perception in large cortical RFs, but synchronizes in time with RGC and V1 foveally aligned new spikes, similar to the short duration metacontrast stimuli that append to latent perceptual spikes, as stated earlier in this chapter.

A camera's film exposed for 100 msec shows a smear of a baseball's motion across the film. However, overlap of motion sensitive M layers and resolution sensitive P layers in the LGN may reduce this motion smear due to serial retinotopic maps with little spatial convergence, which reduce z spike rate as the baseball crosses the field of view.[193] For rapid

---

[192] Gregori-Grgic, R., Balderi, M., de Sperati, C. (2011) PLoS One 6:e17079; this experiment measured a faster relative reflex time of subconscious compared to conscious speed discrimination.

[193] Burr, D. (1980) Nature 284:164, found that 160 msec of target motion produced better target resolution than 40 msec. Hypothetically, with target speed constrained, longer target motion stimulates convergent neurons so that synchronized z spike output results from distinguishable x-y spacing. Frequent updates of target location also improves smooth pursuit accuracy in Osborne et.al. (2005), op. cit.

stimulus movements across the field of view, motion smear may be due to both receptor persistence and long-lasting plexiform graded potentials from short stimulus durations. Here, spikes emitted commensurate with the rate of motion across the retina, act as a temporal strobe so that spikes that have survived successive stages of filtering, blip shorter instants of correlated retinal x-y movement into perceptual continuity, than are in initial high RGC spike rates incurred by smearing motion.[194] Convergent M RGCs must be instrumental for this transient response, so that what is a continuous firing caused by stimulus speed, is perceived with little spatial blur, as described in Burr (1980). Fast recurrent inhibition on inputs may reduce spatial integration of temporally convergent spikes from large RF areas. With multiple stages of convergent x-y summation that reduce spike rate, the fixed emission time of the z spike, and the long interval between spikes re-emitted at late cortical stages, creates less perceived blur of mixed feature and motion inputs on the same convergent neuron.

Spikes move the z location of both slow motion at high retinal resolution, and rapid motion that smears due to lagging retinal potentials and the low resolution that may result from the spatial and temporal convergence on peripheral neurons. While rapid motion transmits the sensation of x-y smear, slower motion over a longer distance and time reduces spike rates successively at serial synapses. At convergent neurons in V5, the low rate of z spikes re-emitted as strobed blips of x-y motion, reduces the

---

[194] Spike temporal precision at retina, as in Greschner et al., is maintained by the precise temporal synchronies of spatially summating M system spikes at cortical synapses. Large numbers of cortical synapses in large cortical RFs, can have high temporal precision that accrue from the rapid movement of a stimulus over a large x-y span.

smear sustained by M RGC spikes, so preventing a persistent perceptual blur.

Do neuronal RFs in V1 mediate perceived fixational stability, or do reemitted z spikes create this perception? Tremor moves image edges across the edges of foveal cone RFs. As anatomically apparent, many midget RGC RFs converge within the bounds of larger binocular V1/V2 simple cell RFs. However, the size of a V1 RF and the location of the boundary where a stimulatory edge elicits a response, varies with differing experimental conditions.[195] FEMs across cone RF edges that map to aligned P cell RFs in V1, emit temporally summated spikes (*Fig. 3.3*), to give a temporary increase in V1 RF size.[196] While V1 RFs minimized in area may jitter with FEMs,[197] the spike rate reemitted by simple cells is less than

---

[195] As previously described, rods and cones input on the same M RGC, which responds to incremental motion during fixation. Gur, M. & Snodderly, D. (1997) Vis. Res. 37:257 record motion-sensitive V1 cells (from M RGCs) by 1) not recording from the 4C beta layer, where foveal P cells that mediate FEM facilitated visual stability input to V1, and 2) moving a stimulus bar at speeds that range to 4 deg/sec, compared to 2-3 deg/sec in Motter & Poggio, op. cit. Chap. One. RF size, and thus RF stability, may vary, as will emitted spike rate, with stimulus luminance, contrast, size and shape, also with prolonged stimulus fixation and spike recording delay (Kara & Reid, op. cit. Chap. One). Without raw data, one must state that small experimental differences aggregate statistically so that Motter & Poggio measure a significant probability of stability of large V1 RFs.

[196] Kara & Reid, Lind et al., op. cit. Chap. One. Averaging spikes over time increases RF size and stability.

[197] Gur, M. & Snodderly, D. (1987) Vis. Res. 27:2081 discuss the induced increase in size of V1 RFs caused by FEMs. To minimize V1 RFs, stimulus size is reduced to create the highest V1 spike rates, also the target is synchronized with retinal motion so that the target is always roughly centered in the RGC RF. The closer edges of smaller V1 RFs jitter as they sustain spikes associated with FEMs. Tang, Y., Saul, A., Gur, M., Goel, S., Wong. E., Ersoy, B., Snodderly, D. (2007) J. Neurophys. 97:3439 explicitly demonstrate the adjustable conditions that reduce spike rate of cells in larger, aligned, convergent V1 RFs (containing more interacting cells), induced by uncompensated FEMs.

half the LGN cell input rate in the same x-y aligned RF.[198] Here, the endurance of proximal-distal aligned z spikes is perceived x-y image stability.[199] P cell temporal summation may result from tremor that stimulates the dual edges of adjoining cone RFs (human tremor between 80-40 Hz has a range that approximates 7-15 sec of arc vs. the 30 seconds of arc diameter of small cones).[200] Microsaccades, at 2-4 Hz, entrain a slow 2-4 Hz rhythm in V1,[201] but this is too infrequent for high resolution and may actually reboot RGCs for proximal-distal z synchronies. Upon fixation on a visual scene, gamma rhythms are induced in V1.[202] V1 gamma rhythms are also inducible without FEM input,[203] so do not require stable RGC spike rates. V1 RFs jitter due to tremor if minimized by stimulus manipulation (V1 RFs were measured to vary about .2 degrees wide at one degree of foveal eccentricity,[204] while recently measured V1 RFs vary in width over .04-.17 degrees at .5

---

[198] Alonso et al., op. cit. Chap. One; a substantially reduced spike rate is true under stimulated and unstimulated conditions in cats.

[199] Kjaer et al., Motter & Poggio, Westheimer & McKee, all op. cit. Chap. One; also van Ee & Erkelens, op. cit.

[200] Eizenman et al., op. cit. Chap. One. Ko, H., Snodderly, D., Poletti, M. (2016) Vis. Res. 122:93 assert that physiologically significant tremor is between 40 and 80 Hz; they also concur with the previous findings of Eizenman and Spauschus et al., op. cit. Tremor amplitude declines as its frequency increases, so may be interpreted as noise.

[201] Ito, J., Maldonado, P., Grun, S. (2013) Front. Sys. Neurosci. 7:1.

[202] Friedman-Hill, S., Maldonado, P., Gray, C. (2000) Cereb. Cort. 10:1105; Cardin, J., Palmer, L., Contreras, D. (2005) J. Neuro. 25:5339.

[203] Bastos, D., Briggs, F., Alitto, H., Mazur, G., Usrey, W. (2014) J. Neurosci. 34:7639; LGN frequencies that input to V1 in alert monkey range over 15-30 Hz, below the 30-100 Hz gamma activity innate to visual cortex and in retinal tremor frequencies.

[204] In macaque cortex, Hubel & Wiesel (1974), op. cit. Chap. One, measured with a single electrode.

degree of eccentricity).²⁰⁵ Temporal and spatial summation of z spikes binocularly integrates aligned monocular inputs. While experimenters may require that V1 RF shifts have mechanisms for 2D image stability, here a cortical video screen is not perceived, but latently reemitted z spikes are perceived, with no x-y RF information. 'Information' here is defined by anatomical label, not a presumed temporal spike code. Identical z spikes are filtered through identical modules distributed throughout V1 cortex. Spatial filtering by modular circuits steers z spikes to specific clusters of IT cells that signal 'category' and synchronize with proximal features in any part of the visual field.

How the relative size and/or jitter of V1 RFs is affected by the amplitude and frequency of FEMs is a subject for analysis at the resolution limits of current technology, with statistical inferences that increase precision only in individual trials, but not in trials averaged over time.²⁰⁶ As discussed earlier, the coordinates of image edges are anatomically defined by foveal RFs that are always at (0,0); here straight least-time light rays are the actual physical reference that impedance match RF and external image edges, to orient and z stabilize perceptually.

In keeping with the impedance match hypothesis detailed in this book, a V1 cell responds univariantly to all receptors in its RF:²⁰⁷ a large proportion of V1 simple cells respond to absolute disparity (a binocular cell's correlation of the monocular spatial posi-

---

[205] McFarland, S., Bondy, A., Cumming, G., Butts., D. (2014) Nature Comm. 5:4605, measured with a planar multi-electrode array.

[206] Tang et al., op. cit.; McFarland, J., Cumming, B., Butts, D. (2016) J. Neurosci. 36:6225.

[207] Li et al., op. cit. Chap. One.

tions of the same image edge), spatial frequency, orientation of a stimulus bar,[208] and even stimuli that are not in natural scenes.[209] This is conventionally called multiplexing, but here, identical z spikes with no disparity, spatial frequency, or orientation information, respond to all data. An increase in spike rate is by convention, a sign of a desirable stimulus feature. But high binocular spike rates result from large absolute disparities; these 'false matches' dominate responses in aggregated trials, but how a precise stereo perception computes from pooled error responses is unknown.[210] High spike rates from matched spatial absolute disparities must also temporally synchronize at specific V1 cells, to reemit onward spikes that synchronize at V2 cells.

While absolute disparity is measured by V1 binocular response to monocular stimulations by the same edge, V2 cells respond to relative disparity, the relative position between two feature edges. Because two edges are a larger part of the visual field, spatial convergence of V1 afferents occurs in V2. Only 10% of V2 cells rapidly reemit from V1 projections, other V2 cells summate more slowly.[211] Latent V2 relative disparity is perceptually stable, with perceived 3D depth and stereoacuity, qualities due to

---

[208] Prince, S., Pointon, A., Cumming, B., Parker, A. (2002) J. Neurophys. 87:191; in this experiment, precision is lost by pooling the responses of 20 trials of the same cell at each of 7-9 disparities of a 2 second stimulus. Input/output convergence/divergence synaptic anatomy and details of reemission timing are also not specified.

[209] Read, J. & Cumming, B. (2007) Nature Neurosci. 10:1322.

[210] De Angelis, G. & Cumming, B. (2001) Ann. Rev. Neurosci. 24:203, Tanabe, S., Haefner, R., Cumming, B. (2011) J. Neurosci. 31:8295; any single V1 cell's responses to different stereogram disparities will elicit an average single and population response of great complexity.

[211] El-Shamayleh, Y., Kumbhani, R., Dhruv, N., Movshon, J. (2013) J. Neurosci. 33:16594; wider APs may cause more rapid summations.

relative spike latencies in larger V2 RFs, which are invariant to the vergence angle or focal distance of the eyes that V1 cells respond to.[212] Finer relative disparity discriminations occur in V4, where V2 projects. The integration of larger relative disparities requires more neural convergence, but stimulated spike rates in V4 are not lower than in V1.[213] In fact, a higher spike rate which the observer perceives as an error response may not signal error in the responsive neuron. Because V4 is part of the repeated 2D neural circuitry necessary for stereoscopic tuning, it requires fine temporal resolution by high reemitted z spike rates, which may integrate aligned with unaligned 'error' spike rates. The 3D precision and stability of perception in IT cortex, is enabled by a precise, convergent z synchronization.

Up to this point, several hypotheses have been put forth to explain fixational stability; among them, that z spikes reemit from precise dual input spike times from tremor, which converge x-y labeled neurons but emit a spatially stable 1D z spike; that the fovea is egocentrically stable because it is neurally hard-wired at the same (0,0) point no matter where it saccades; that least-time light rays and neural spike paths transiently align external edges with retinotopically mapped RF boundaries via spikes timed by shifting foveal RGCs, which temporally synchronize at spatially convergent synapses; that larger V1

---

[212] Westheimer (1979) op. cit. Chap. One; Cumming, B. & Parker, A. (1999) J. Neurosci. $\underline{19}$:5602; the fused stereo perception comprises Panum's area. Tanabe, S. & Cumming, B. (2008) J. Neurosci. $\underline{28}$:11304 compare V1 vs. V2 RFs, firing rates and other properties.

[213] Umeda, K., Tanabe, S., Fujita, I. (2007) J. Neurophys. $\underline{98}$:241; Shiozaki, H., Tanabe, S., Doi, T., Fujita, I. (2012) J. Neurosci. $\underline{32}$:3830. The error bars measured from successive trials for the same relative disparity discrimination are very small, indicating that short precise spike intervals are necessary for fine discriminations.

RFs create a visual stability, due to synapses that spatially converge inputs from smaller receptor RFs; and that shifting receptors stimulate a latent, persistent perception of both a 3D image and stability, integrated in the same convergent z spikes in IT cortex, which have a delayed, phase-locked synchrony with the shifting frequency of retinal FEMs.

One can model a neurophysiological mechanism that integrates these alternatives with the following: fixational tremor acts as a precise timer of edge-stimulated spikes, which emit only at the same repeatable image edge position in a receptor's RF.[214] This precise spike timing conveys the same x-y location of the external edge relative to other edges, triggered by the simultaneous timing of tremor over the whole retina. In higher organisms, identical tremor-triggered spikes (with no x-y coding) align with previous spatially convergent, long-duration cortical z spikes, from a stable external edge, transiently (0,0) aligned with cone RF edges oscillating due to retinal tremor. It is the shift-induced, x-y synchronization of foveal RGC z spikes in RF-aligned, least-time paths to the LGN or SC (0,0) locations that is perceived over convergent time with both x-y precision and external edge stability. With large shifts in retinal response due to large saccades, the spikes generated by the new target attach to the z spikes from the previously fixated target without coded x-y information, to give the perception of peripheral image stability due to synchronous z locations and times emitted in early retinotopic stages, which endure latently without x-y labels in distal IT cortex. Experiments show a re-

---

[214] Greschner et al. op. cit. Chap. One; Sincich et al. (2009), op. cit.; find that spike rate emitted from the convergent neuron is very sensitive to the location of the stimulated photoreceptor in the RF.

sponse bias in foveal V1 to not only straight ahead, but angularly oblique targets.[215] Here, this bias is because the fovea is always at anatomical (0,0) no matter where targeted. Absolute x-y coordinates of retinal RFs vis-a-vis image edges are not temporally coded by identical z spikes; synchronous z durations are stable, impedance-matched, aligned references.

The fixational instability of minimized binocular RFs in V1 to monocular disparities,[216] is consistent here with hardwired foveal maps at SC, LGN and V1, which define an anatomical (0,0) by FEM jitter that generates spikes at foveal RFs. As stated, synapses in higher cortical centers reemit from synchronized, contrast-stimulated spikes; the synchronization of latent z spikes at convergent synapses does not require encoded x-y coordinates, of the image edge or of the foveal RF. Edges that generate synchronous RGC spikes align with previous reemitted cortical z spikes of longer latencies in V1, V2, V4 and IT, due to neural convergence within the same distal RF. The z spike endurance reemits as an unshifting temporal percept of jittery anatomical 2D x-y RFs.

The precision of RGC spike timing vis-a-vis stimulus position, increases with edge contrast,[217] an indication that spikes are not a code of contrast in the image, but that contrast-timed spikes abruptly synchronize the emission of spikes at convergent synapses. Otherwise, imprecise timing, or bending of the light ray passing the external edge, would smear

---

[215] Durand, J-P., Trotter, Y., Celebrini, S. (2010) Neuron 66:126; here the least-time z axis is always at (0,0) in the fovea, SC, LGN and V1.

[216] Gur & Snodderly (1987) op. cit., Cumming & Parker op. cit.; these deviations in fixational disparity (by foveal RFs) that cause V1 cell RFs to shift, are much smaller than in Motter & Poggio, op. cit. Chap. One.

[217] Berry et al. op. cit.

image location, with concomitant perceptual blur and distortion. While the external observer sees retinal receptors that blur x-y imagery over the time of the perceptual moment, the subject sees only precise least-time z spikes stimulated by light rays at image edges, in which slow, noisy spikes at the wrong time and x-y location do not summate or average over time for latent perception. The neural circuits at each level of the early visual hierarchy are organized so that orthogonal x-y synchronized inputs emit onward z spikes, to endure distally as sequentially synchronized z perceptions.

The light ray and the retinal response to edge contrast, stimulate the shortest, fastest path via the FEM shifts of orthogonal receptors, to corresponding V1 locations retinotopically aligned with the external image. This match from points in the visual field, via z spikes to object and facial recognition areas of IT cortex, is synchronized over z distance and time by reemission of spikes from serial arrays of synapses. As described in the next chapter, the synchronous existence of identical z spikes at RGC and IT cortex, rather than information coded by sequential spikes that is cortically decoded, allows peripheral sensory information to be a latent z perception.

Perceptual stability created by anatomical and temporal summation of spikes easily adapts neural mechanisms that respond to novel input, as shown in the Murakami & Cavanagh experiments mentioned earlier in this chapter. The transient stability of the Necker cube illusion, here does not depend on information transfer that integrates over time in perceptual cortex. The switchable percept may be due to phase-locked relationships of spikes in cortical neurons that fatigue, or adapt, from sustained spikes from the same monocular images, which shifts the neuronal routes to univariant neurons of longer latency.[218] This shifts one binocular cortical 3D perception to another, temporally synchronous with the same RGC sustained spikes stimulated by the dual 2D retinal images.

This adaptability of cortical neurons is relevant to the binocular perception of stereo 3D depth in random dot stereograms, used to record absolute disparities of cells in V1, as discussed a few pages ago. The predominance of high firing rates in multiple cells at non-zero disparities is thought to be a population code that is decoded as the perceived binocular 3D image. Monocular edges necessarily emit spikes that stimulate a population of binocularly responsive V1 neurons that reemit varying rates, most are called 'false matches'.[219] However, if V1 cells that respond to absolute disparity of the same edge are recorded in a short temporal window in response to a single vergence angle of the eyes and with one stereogram presentation, then the binocularly re-emitted spikes from the neurally equidistant, FEM-synchronized monocular edges should be perceived as stereopsis when spikes converge on V2 cells. Perceived 3D depth is a result of binocular cells that respond to monocular retinal z latencies that average around 60 msec, with orthogonal interocular edge-matched timing delays tolerated to 15-20 msec.[220] Changes in absolute disparities or changes in vergence angle induce changes in maximal firing rate in the same binocular V1 cell. Binocular re-

---

[218] Cumming & Parker, op. cit., also, lowering binocular disparity cues causes bistability of the stereo image.

[219] Marr, D. & Poggio, T. (1979) Proc. Roy. Soc. B Biol. Sci. 204:301.

[220] Read & Cumming, op. cit. Chap. One; Trotter, Y., Celebrini, S., Stricanne, B., Thorpe, S. (1996) J. Neurophys. 76:2872; Busettini, C., Miles, F., Krauzlis, R. (1996) J. Neurophys. 75:1392.

sponses of longer latency, ranging above 150 msec in humans, are due to the motor delay to accommodate lenses and binocularly verge dual retinal images as a single image, and for perceptual 3D fusion of varied distances and disparities induced by equidistant 2D random dots in stereogram images. Experiments are being designed to perhaps explain the indiscriminate population responses of binocular V1 neurons to multiple disparities and dynamic stereograms during the fixation period, which may result in less heterogeneous data, of low statistical significance as currently analyzed. Here, RGC RFs, synchronized by FEMs, sequence emitted z times at serial x-y convergent synapses that retain precision from coinciding monocular spatial disparity RFs and from temporally matched spikes at binocular cells from the same edge. A virtual, perceived 3D x-y-z synchrony results from neurally aligned external image edges that stimulate repeated high spike rates in 2D arrays of V1, V2, V4 and IT, a precision that is not in averaged V1 transient and sustained population responses to edge crossings.[221]

The fastest neural route for a train of spikes is repeatable, that is, invariant compared with slower routes, because divergent routes may vary randomly in length. What could be a normal distribution of routes and times is narrowed; repetitious inputs reinforce the least-time route with the fewest synapses. If synchronized inputs are timed in parallel to emit new z spikes at synapses, the correct perception of external temporal sequence and spatial order is preserved, because slower divergent spikes are inhibited, so do not synchronize peripheral with perceptual areas. The least-time route is experimentally reproducible because it represents a

---
[221] Kagan, I., Gur, M., Snodderly, D. (2008) J. Vision $\underline{8}$:1.

learned, synaptically facilitated neural path. Spike timing dependent synaptic facilitation and depression, forms of neural learning, require a correlation of less than 20 msec between convergent spikes to causally modify a synapse in V1 cortex.[222] Learning is a sustained effect of spikes at the same synapses, which in binocular V1 cells synchronize due to equal wiring distances and latencies of monocular spikes stimulated by the same edge. Adapting to prisms to perceive visual stability of images, must also result from synchronized learning by synapses.

Prisms modify the perception of image stability after saccades by altering where the target in the image inputs onto the hard-wired retinotopic map vis-a-vis the fovea. Over a period, which can be more than a month for left-right reversing prisms, less for wedge prisms, the subject adapts to this awkward positioning of target versus retinotopic fovea, so that motor responses gradually become accurate.[223] Exaggerated spike responses at contrasty image edges, as outlined earlier in this chapter, align retinotopic, motor and proprioceptive somatotopic maps. A prism-shifted target alters the x-y location of highest sensory inputs on these repeated maps, requiring sensory adaptation and modification of motor outputs.[224] Sensory adaptation to increased inputs in parallel retinotopic maps, can shift neuronal input-output relationships without completely rewiring the SC map. Shifted synapses in parallel retinotopic areas are stimulated by this sensory target

---

[222] Meliza, C. & Dan, Y. (2006) Neuron 49:183.

[223] Sekiyama, K., Miyauchi, S., Imaruoka, T., Egusa, J., Tashiro, T. (2000) Nature 407:374, map MRI brain responses to prisms.

[224] Block, H. & Bastian, A. (2012) Neuropsychologia 50:1766; the cerebellum is required for motor-reaching adaptation to changed target location and distance.

shift, which respond to newly synchronous inputs; synaptic learning occurs with repetition. The dominance of the new sensory learning reroutes inputs to the hardwired retinotopically aligned motor outputs from the SC, to create a new awareness of accurate target location, but with a probable longer latency due to the longer route.

This adaptation to shifted input is not due to a looping error signal, but a latent awareness of target discrepancy on the foveal area of the V1 map that dominates, to shift subliminal retinotopic plasticity in other areas. Spikes have no x-y data, but increased spikes alter synaptic density at a shifted anatomic location, which with repetition at that x-y location, learn a rewired foveal area on the map.

Let's revisit how perception of a visually tracked sinusoidally moving target that is subsequently occluded, can synchronize reaching with target position. Within the 150 msec perceptual moment, factors such as motor neural and muscle activation delays, feedback from proprioception to somatosensory cortex and the neural activation delays of visual perception in larger distal cortical RFs, synchronize proximal-distal locations/times so that the subject perceives that there are no delays. To dissociate sensory delays that fuse perceptually, from spike latencies due to motor movements that follow predictable sinusoidal target motion, one can increase visual cognitive feedback delay to 200 msec or more.[225] Retinotopic alignment of 2D maps keep perception anatomically oriented despite increased convergent latencies within larger RFs to give x-y-z spatially and temporally integrated percepts. Re-

---

[225] Miall, R., Weir, V., Wolpert, D., Stein, J. (1993) J. Motor Behav. 25:203; Rohde, M., Greiner, L., Ernst, M. (2014) J. Vis. 14:article 4.

petitive motor and sensory learning at convergent synapses, causes the initial subjective perception of prism or other artificially-induced delay, to gradually reduce the perception of spatial dissonance. However, induced delays worsen motor performance, so that subjects increase training duration, suggesting that anatomical circuits shift, as mentioned in the last paragraph. Normally, evoked spike latencies from auditory, touch and vision stimuli have highest magnitudes that range from 90 to 130 msec in the corresponding cortical areas;[226] these sustained spikes overlap durations at temporal integration areas such as the multisensory SC,[227] where sensory inputs summate to emit onward perceptual spikes.

In delayed feedback experiments, a psychometric sense of maximal perceived simultaneity is measured while the subject is trained with a light flash delay of 150 msec; if 100 msec is added to this delay, the percept of maximal simultaneity adjusts, to an added duration of 23 to 44 msec relative to the initial percept.[228] This temporal summation at the SC (and LGN) surface must be orthogonal, to be so short in duration relative to the total 250 msec perception. The continuously reemitted, enduring z spikes lengthen the perceptual moment but within that 150 to 250 msec, is a 45 msec orthogonal precision at x-y SC and LGN surfaces.[229] Thus no para-

---

[226] Rohde M. & Ernst, M. (2013) Front. Psychol. 03:599.

[227] Meredith, M., Nemitz, J., Stein, B. (1987) J. Neurosci. 7:3215.

[228] Stetson, C., Cui, X., Montague, R., Eagleman, D. (2006) Neuron 51:651. The 23-44 msec precision measured, overlaps the LGN temporal integration period of 33 msec stated earlier in this chapter. This FEM-synchronized precision must occur at initial layers of synapses.

[229] Schmid, M., Mrowka, S., Turchig, J., Saunders, J., Wilke, M., Peters, A., Ye, F., Leopold, D. (2010) Nature 466:373; the subliminal state is true of spikes in the parallel SC and LGN stages of the visual system.

dox exists if sensory inputs at these early stages are subliminal; due to spikes that temporally summate within 45 msec, long-duration z spikes reemit, for a 150-250 msec perceptual moment in distal stages. The result is consistent with integrative cortical latencies of 150 msec from visual, somatosensory and auditory inputs, which perceptually synchronize with emitted instants of time at labeled sensory receptors. However, perceptual delays over 150 msec uncouple the perceptual moment from sensory inputs and/or motor outputs, to increase motor inaccuracy to predictable target motion.[230]

Firing activity in SC neurons contains no conventionally measured information code of simple stimuli, even after 100 msec of sustained or reentrant firing from stimulus onset.[231] This is consistent with sensory APs that do not encode information in spike rate over time, rather, specific receptor types and labeled circuits within convergent RFs select image features anatomically. Others find that synaptic output information increases, despite the reduction in spike rate, due to precisely timed output spikes resulting from temporally coincident inputs.[232] This increased precision of output spikes due to temporally synchronous inputs, is the key to the integrated idea here that z spikes reemit outputs at temporally and spatially convergent cortical synapses that per-

---

[230] Miall & Jackson, op. cit.

[231] Krauzlis & Dill, op. cit.; as stated here, spikes possess transient z-location, not image information; still, temporal spike correlations are an indirect measure of cortical sensing of retinal information; redefinition of spike function, without conventional information, is required.

[232] LGN output spikes are interpreted to increase in information due to the close timing (<30 msec) of input spikes necessary to reemit output spikes, in Dan, Y., Alonso, J., Usrey, W., Reid, R. (1998) Nature Neurosci. $\underline{1}$:501; Reinagel P. & Reid, R. (2000) J. Neurosci. $\underline{20}$:5392; Sincich et al. (2009) op. cit. Chap, One.

ceptually synchronize with peripheral retinal x-y information. Long intervals between spikes may persist perceptually over time along the z axis, akin to phosphors stimulated at a high frame rate across a video screen's x-y plane. Because z spikes have no spatial information, smear reduces with high rates of newly appended retinal spikes, as with a looming fastball. One may perceive what are ordinarily subliminally shifting inputs, due to least-time z synchronies of aligned foveal inputs (*Fig. 3.3*) and the convergent sequence of incremental motion detected in M RGCs. Adjacent lagging inputs actually may augment temporally summated reemission to increase V1 foveal resolution. Finally, the longer intervals between V5 z spikes due to summated M RGC spatial and temporal convergence over the extent of the perceptual moment, give the perception of apparent motion without a percept of blur; distal z spikes do not transmit x-y smearing of motion from adjacent receptors, which is also subliminal.[233]

From a different cognitive perspective, why does an organism's sense of visual stability not require continuously referenced x,y,z coordinates? We have stated here that an absolute external or internal reference is not necessary for egocentric visual stability. Some interpret this egocentricity as relativistic. But saccades on the SC's retinotopic surface are absolute distances.[234] At first glance, a sense of ego-

---

[233] Morgan, M. (1980) Phil. Trans. R. Soc. Lond. B $\underline{290}$:137 discusses two neural areas that mediate apparent motion, with latencies at 32 and 128 ms; the first area may be the LGN, which is implicated in video frame integration, and the latter area may be V5 cortex. Some investigators interpret 32 msec as a short perceptual moment.

[234] That the SC uses absolute orthogonal coordinates may be necessary for external edges to be accurately sensed by fixed-time z spikes emitted at RGC RF edges. These psychophysical experiments are in van Dam, L., Hawellek, D., Ernst, M. (2013) J. Vis. $\underline{13}$:article 26.

centric stability under unpredictable environmental conditions, needs to be metabolically 'on' at all times, to maintain a continuous sense of visual stability. But greater efficiency results when egocentric stability does not use energy all the time to continuously stabilize reference coordinates from vision or the VOR, but maintains a resting noisy slow firing rate, as is characteristic of P cells, which respond at a high rate to transient 'errors' in the position of the fixation target on the retina.[235] So any fixation on any target has an absolute, anatomically defined (0,0) point that is always on center; a high spike rate is not necessary to code image or foveal (0,0) coordinates.

Essential to the understanding of the duration of the perceptual moment, is that this time is not an autonomous sliding window, but is created by the continuous duration of each serially reemitted spike. A retinal spike starts a least-time clock, which ends if serially summated z spikes do not end in IT cortex within 120-150 msec. The continuous reemission of spikes, during a fixation of a similar duration, create the indivisibility of the perceptual moment. Over a long time these recurrent z spike durations become the continuous time commonly called consciousness.

The sustained retinal output resulting from a long fixation, after the least-time spikes that result in IT categorization of an object, must input as delayed synaptic summations that integrate contextual detail about the object. Divergent spike routing that results in delayed reemission could surface as dreams that are not ordinarily perceived in the presence of

---
[235] Laughlin, S. & Sejnowski (2003) Science 301:1870; they conclude that about 50% of power used by the brain is steady state maintenance of neuronal metabolism and resting spike rates.

strong, synchronized sensory input; or emerge as correlations of combined thoughts known as intuition or an imprecise 'gist'.[236] The delayed percepts of context in the largest RFs, are enabled by the larger dendritic fields and much greater quantities of synapses of these latter cortical areas.[237] The spatial and temporal convergence of spikes at these synapses, in overlapping and more diffuse RF boundaries, emit spikes from the same synapses facilitated during learning, causing recurrent and/or delayed imaginary meanderings, daydreams, subtle thoughts and resurgent memories that can dominate sensory inputs impinging in real time. Also, the tiling of dendritic fields from neighboring receptors can both integrate inputs over larger spatial areas (as a gist, detailed context or intuition) and also enable precise timing and spatial discriminations at synapses simultaneously stimulated.[238]

In this chapter, the author has stated several hypotheses to explain persistent image stability. None of these alternatives create defined spatial coordinates in larger cortical RFs from which self motion can be discriminated from external motion. Two of the hypotheses seem more important--convergent egocentricity resulting from shifting inputs on the same foveal (0,0) anatomical center, and least-time spike and neural paths through temporally synchronized, transiently aligned external and RF edge crossings. FEM-synchronized spikes emit from im-

---

[236] Lamme V., Roelfsema, P. (2000) Trends Neurosci. 23:571; Sugase et al., op. cit.; delayed spikes can also synchronize peripheral details correlated with categorization of a facial type, such as its expression or specific identity.

[237] Elston, G. (2003) Neurosci. 117: 213.

[238] See Lund et al., op. cit. Chap. One, and Dan et al., op. cit., for discussion of overlapping RFs between pairs of neurons.

age edge-crossings that reemit, enduring in z time as they converge to specific synapses in larger perceptual RFs, creating a perception of externally integrated features that are externally stable due to proximal-distal synchronous duration of 1D z spikes that mediate the perceptual moment. The hypotheses discussed can be tested to exclude others. However, integration and analysis of the proposed mechanisms increase our understanding of synergistic visual image stability.

CONCLUSIONS

1) The first chapter demonstrated that an action potential reliably moves a location from an orthogonal 2D surface, as a third z dimension. This chapter shows that the temporal durability of the reemitted z spike enables the simultaneous presence of aligned z spikes via wired connections between repeated 2D maps. The sequential z spikes generated from the same edge over fixational time, acquire a synchronous timing property over neural distance, which, due to identical non-informational spikes at the same repeated 2D x-y location over z distance, make these locations z equivalent.

2) A necessary consequence of the hypothesis of z equivalence, in which sustained 1D z spikes are present both at the sensory periphery and in cortical perception areas at the same time, at serial retinotopic locations during fixation, is that the phase synchronization of z spikes transiently at proximal-distal synapses integrates convergent reemitted latent perceptions at cortical surfaces with current informational stimulation at sensory surfaces.

3) While spike speed is important to quickly update cortex about peripheral events, under sustained spiking rates, the coordinated match of spike speed with spike repetition rate and z distance between x-y topographically mapped synapses in arrays, allows phase-locking. This repeated emission of identical z spikes (of the same label), makes the physical 3D temporal and spatial interval between equivalently mapped 2D arrays, virtual when summated into continuous perception, due to the phase-locked property of 1D identical spikes that move z location sequentially, at repeated, RF-aligned 2D arrays.

4) Rather than neural loops that feed visual targeting information to a comparison point, with concomitant feedback delays that result in lagged inaccuracy, spikes emitted in response to high-contrast edges keep RF boundaries aligned in repeated retinotopically mapped arrays. The orthogonal properties of adjacent sensory-motor maps correct slight sensory-motor dislocations in msec time as sustained z spikes traverse them. The 1D reemitted z spikes, with no coded x-y error except in spike rate, stabilize via a latent z perceptual moment without a delayed comparison of a latent x-y image on the retinal x-y image.

5) The amplitude of retinal tremor in primates matches the boundary-edges of a foveal receptor RF with the high-contrast stimulus edge; this is evidence for impedance matching of external edges and dimensions of receptors. Due to a hard-wired fovea on the SC map that has the same (0,0) anatomically mapped coordinates no matter where saccadically targeted, and also due to a similar magnitude of spike response to both exogenous stimulus movements and endogenous retinal movements, remapping of fixational foveal x-y locations to stabi-

lize the perception of external x-y image locations does not occur. This egocentric stability occurs without adding or subtracting reference x-y coordinates from (0,0); convergent 1D z spikes therefore are a stable percept that lasts over time without averaging shifting x-y information.

6) Eye movements, most typically tremor that crosses receptor boundaries and stimulus edges, generate 2D-synchronized spikes. The repeated, abrupt emission of spikes from RGCs creates temporally convergent synchronies at later synapses. Which synapses emit in response to synchronous inputs does not matter, the filtered spikes that endure determine which retinal x-y inputs have synchronized with latent perception. This egocentric stability uses as a reference light rays themselves, which are not only straight, but couple or impedance match an external photon least-time with edge-stimulated spikes that take a rapidly-reemitted path through convergent synapses.

Where Did the Time Go?

What is time? We know that it has a lasting accumulative quantity, but if we try to be locally specific, we find that it is transient. Time is a necessary accompaniment of any spatial dimension, though conceived generically as a single time dimension; space, by its extensive properties requires time to traverse. The directionality of abstract time can be ambiguous, because physical laws that use time squared, are consistent with both negative and positive time. In Chapter Two, time was shown to be mapped to spatial locations in the hippocampus, so that memory, as time, can move forward and backward in spatial sequence, though the observer senses memory in one direction due to the observer's initial birth time, which is the obvious base for a causal sequence of memories. Linear time is coextensive with linear spatial dimensions, as shown in *Fig. 2.1*, so that experienced time can cycle backward, but not forward, from the current time. A time point is measurable at any of many equivalent points, serially marked with different symbols on a time-line. Time points can also accumulate, rather than be serially independent. Characteristic frequency decreases and wavelength increases, with high atomic frequencies that aggregate time lags into a lower frequency for the whole crystal. Also, the frequencies of alloyed metals superpose as the dimensional frequency of an organ pipe. In general, as spatial area or volume increases, characteristic wavelength increases, accruing more standard time units within the resonant or synchronous periodicity of the material.

In brain physiology, various parameters, such as spike averages over various windows of time, and rate codes and frequency codes, are measured at stationary electrode locations. Area voltages recorded from stimulus-evoked spikes in multiple neurons with a surface electrode on the skull, called evoked potentials (EPs), are averaged with repetition of the same stimulus, to reduce individual latency and magnitude variability. Here EP spike 'latency' means time from stimulation to maximal spike response. EPs at multiple cortical locations are measured as the EEG. Transient spikes averaged at each electrode produce the waves of voltage, called oscillations, in the EEG; if moving APs at an EEG electrode do not add at a latent time at that place, the oscillations should average as a flat line. Reentrant (or recurrent) oscillations can be measured at several cortical locations in serial time.

Phase-locking can be shown, by recording the synchronized spikes firing at the same point in the oscillatory cycle, from the same group of neurons at the same cortical location. This coordinated firing may lag or advance the highest amplitude of spike rates during the cycle, depending upon stimulus intensity, stimulus orientation and other experimental conditions.[239] Synchronization varies with time according to mental activity, so that it can alternately desynchronize, or synchronize at different frequencies at specific cortical locations.[240] These synchronized frequencies indicate a repetitious correlation in time of spikes between cortical areas of the brain that have specific perceptual or integrative properties. Wavelength increases as distance between those synchronized areas increases.[241] Both large scale frequency, and local phase lags within the synchronized frequency, can vary with electrode location relative to a reference topographical location.

Why do the conditions of identical spikes in labeled neurons and z locus equivalence, described in the first chapter, scale to many neurons, so that spikes fire between distant 2D surfaces in temporal synchrony, bypassing the additive properties of causal sequential time over increased distance? One clue is that a neuron's length is necessary to connect non-adjacent surfaces; spikes need to associate areas, not just with sequential delay, but when sustained, distant locations at the same time. Is a necessary property of phenomenological perception, given by large scale synchronization at retinotopic surfaces, to be as perceptually correlated as a video screen positioned equidistantly in front of an observer? This simultaneity is similar to findings in

---

[239] Konig, P., Engel, A., Roelfsema, P., Singer, W. (1995) Neural Comp. 7:469.

[240] Varela, F., LaChaux, J-P., Rodriguez, E., Martinerie, J. (2001) Nature Rev. Neurosci. 2:229, review the techniques that validate phase-locked frequencies that increase wavelength with neural distance.

[241] Von Stein, A. & Sarntheim, J. (2000) Int. J. Psychophysiol. 38:301; Fries, P., Neuenschwander, S., Engel, A., Goebel, R., Singer, W. (2001) Nature Neurosci. 4:194.

physics, consistent with perceptual sensation, that demonstrate entanglement in divergent photons; flipping the spin of one photon is 'entangled' in time with the detection of spin-flip in the other photon, over a great spatial distance.[242] Neural synchrony may be a more accessible realm for study of synchronous time than spin-flipping photons. The question remains, does neural synchrony result from sequential physical processes that synthesize a sense of simultaneity, or does causal standardized time emerge from a prior state of synchronous spikes at repeated 2D surfaces? In support of this last alternative, simultaneous sensory correlations have been shown psychophysically to precede the perception of sequence.[243]

An explanation for phase-locked firing at synapses has been proposed. Briefly, correlated spikes converge, summate, and reemit spikes that are even more temporally correlated, due to fast-spiking inhibition by interneurons that stop laggard spikes from summating, therefore sharpening and narrowing the temporal and spatial convergent window for summation at the next synapse.[244] Timely spike convergence at synapses to cause synchronous reemission

---

[242] Entanglement and its validity over distance, are a currently debated issue in physics, see for example Wolf, M., Verstraete, F., Hastings, M., Cirac, J.I. (2008) Phys. Rev. Lett. 100:070502.

[243] Parise, C., Spence, C., Ernst, M. (2012) Curr. Biol. 22:46.

[244] Tamas et al., op. cit. Chap. Three; Cardin, J., Carlen, M., Meletis, K., Knobbish, U., Zhang, F., Deisseroth, K., Tsai, L., Moore, C. (2009) Nature 459:663; Pouille, F. & Scanziani, M. (2001) Science 293:1159. Summation at the pyramidal cell (PYC) soma occurs within 2.4 msec and in its dendritic field over 10 msec. In Vaidya, S. & Johnson, D. (2013) Nature Neurosci. 16:1812, a PYC synchronizes dissimilar dendritic delays, altering the gamma rhythm to the much slower theta rhythm. Milstein, A., Bloss, E., Apostolides, P., Vaidya, S., Dilly, G., Zemelman, G., Magee, J. (2015) Neuron 87:1274 show that rapid summation at synapses preferentially passes high frequencies.

is robust to experimentally induced phase lags or differences in spike latency.[245]

Spikes recorded at maximal distance between the cortical hemispheres, with conduction delays of about 6 msec in cats, synchronize within two oscillations with a zero phase-lag,[246] much faster than in simulated networks of coupled oscillators.[247] Oscillations over time and space synchronize at a single point in time and space due to reciprocal connections with inhibitory time-sharpening circuitry.[248] However, bilateral phase-locking disrupts if the corpus callosum between the hemispheres is cut. Synchronous frequency depends on a neuronal path between the cortical locations recorded and is not due to the shortest physical distance between the locations.[249] The thalamus is thought to be a central emitter of synchronizing spikes, with the same latency to various cortical distances.[250]

The 30-80 Hz low gamma rhythm overlaps tremor frequency in humans of 40-100 Hz that generates

---

[245] Konig, P., Engel, A., Singer, W. (1995) PNAS (USA) 92:290; Konig, P. & Schillen, T. (1991) Neural Comp. 3:155.

[246] Engel, A. Konig, P., Kreitzer, A., Singer, W. (1991) Science 252:1177; Berger, D., Warren, D., Norman, R., Arieli, A., Gruen, S. (2007) Neurocomputing 70:2112; this interhemispheric delay in humans can be 27 msec in myelinated fibers; in Ringo, J., Doty, R., Demeter, S., Simard, P. (1994) Cereb. Cortex 4:331.

[247] Fox, J., Wang, D., Campbell, S., Jayaprakash, C. (2001) Neural Comput. 13:1003.

[248] Distributed oscillations and local synchrony differ, shown in Salinas, E. & Sejnowski, T. (2001) Nature Rev. Neurosci. 2:539.

[249] Csicsuari, J., Jamieson, B., Wise, K., Buzsaki, G. (2003) Neuron 37:311.

[250] Salami, M., Itani, C., Tsumoto, T., Kimura, F. (2003) PNAS (USA) 100:6174.

RGC spikes; this rhythm is generated in PYC circuits and occurs not only in mice but in the local circuits of large primate cortices.[251] As stated in Chapter One, cortical PYC output affects fixational tremor, which causes RGCs to emit spikes; but fixated imagery causes cortical gamma rhythms,[252] a causal circularity that creates debate. In primates viewing an image, phase-locking is already present in the first spikes following a saccade and fixation on the image, with an initial spike latency of ~40 msec to V1 cortex.[253] It is thought that this synchronization indicates initial segregation of image features, or awareness of oriented edges, in convergent simple cell RFs. As stated here, spikes do not code information, nor does synchrony move data. Here, if topographically mapped surfaces phase-lock, identical, mobile z spikes temporally fuse the surfaces.

To expand on this last scenario, synchronization of x-y matched z locations by spikes requires a firing rate and speed synchronized with the approximate distance between the synapses. If synaptic activation of disparate cortical locations occurs at approximately the same time during spike synchronization, the disparate perceptions transiently fuse at the same objective time, enabled by the multiple presence of sustained z spikes during the perceptual moment. Normally, the synchronization of firing at specific cortical areas organizes so that there is no conmingling of sensations, such as in synaesthesia,

---

[251] Buzsaki et al., op. cit. from Chap. One, discuss scale-free oscillation frequencies that are independent of brain size.

[252] Friedman-Hill et al., Cardin et al., op. cit.

[253] Maldonado, P., Babel, C., Singer, W., Rodriguez, E., Berger, D., Grun, S. (2008) J. Neurophys. 100:1523. Phase-locking was measured between nearby neuron pairs. After fixation onset, phase-locking occurs rapidly in V1 but decreases before peak spike rate is achieved.

to create a confused percept of a blue sound. In fact, synchronous firing may be the only way to recognize external image relationships that would otherwise be neural noise. If cortical areas do not synchronize, this is a neural signal that stimulus features are not behaviorally recognized by monkeys as a face.[254] Spikes do not change shape upon synchronization,[255] so cannot be transmitting encoded facial features to a distal location this way.

To examine this topic further, a simple but robust physiological model shows how timing correlations of spikes at synapses, rather than sparse information coded by spikes, accounts for reading cognition, as well as psychophysical phenomena previously described. This model applies in two hierarchical stages, first from fovea to V1, V2 and V4 to assemble components into shapes of letters; and then to the border of IT cortex in an area called the visual word form area (VWFA) that assembles meanings from the components of words and sentences, no matter the size, shape, capitalization or style of the lettering.[256] Initially, the contrasty edges of letters generate spikes from midget RGCs during fixation; neighboring RGCs grouped as an oriented line on the retina, i.e. a '/', emit spikes that simultaneously summate at a V1 oriented simple cell. Further simultaneous convergent summations in larger RFs, emit in response to specific orientations of '/', assemblies such as an 'A'. Still further convergent summations of temporally synchronous spikes re-

---

[254] Tsunoda, K., Yamane, Y., Nishizaki, N., Tanifuji, M. (2001) Nature Neurosci. 4:832. Components of a face that were jumbled for stimulus presentation caused no synchronization, while a meaningfully intact, recognizable face caused widespread cortical synchronization.

[255] Heck, D., Thach, W., Keating. J. (2007) PNAS (USA) 104: 7658.

[256] Dehaene, S. (2009) Reading in the Brain.

spond, in V4 to an assembly of letters, for example the word 'FACE' containing 'A'. Seven to nine letters process in parallel during each reading fixation. These sequential summations, in which the neural distance to convergent synapses in cortical RFs is proportional to the latency of spikes from the retina, couple the successive reduction in spike rates from correlated inputs, with larger RF areas. Synchronized spikes converge at each stage to correlate sequential perceptions with letter, then word groups.

This hierarchy does not require that the contrasty edge information at the retina's receptors be transmitted all the way to cortex, to be perceived as an 'A' in the midst of a paragraph containing the word 'FACE'. A reading fixation and the perceptual moment last long enough for the sustained response to 'A' to be seen during the same fixation as the convergent spatial and temporal correlated spike emitted for 'FACE' in a distally larger RF. Here, fixation-induced spikes do not transmit information over time, but because the emitted time is a fixed instant (as the stimulus edge crossed the receptor), it stays fixed due to the proportional distance/time of a moving spike that convergently synchronizes at each serial synapse. The rapidly moving reemitted spike retains the fixed emission times of input spikes synchronously stimulated by FEMs of the total retina. The static time of the reemitted spike, in effect, is one memory of the synchronized, fixed times of multiple edge-crossing spikes. Simultaneous convergent inputs of component letters that combine as the word 'FACE' will therefore have a much lower post-synaptic spike rate than is possible if spikes reemitted the information of every component letter. Because static times of spikes emitted at each synaptic stage are seen at the same time during fixation, letters, words, and the meanings of words are understood within the typical reading fixation of 300 msec.[257] FEM-induced spikes emit synchronously to summate rapidly at each synaptic stage, so that the convergent 'FACE' synapse and the parallel inputs that temporally correlate due to neighboring words at neighboring synapses, add serial fixed times, or meanings, in larger VWFA RFs.

The spikes that result from synchronized spike responses to neighboring words, temporally and spatially summate at a larger convergent VWFA RF, whose reduced spike emission rate indicates a fixed meaning for the whole word group. If an adjacent word also has an 'A', this is not only spatially and temporally distinct on the retina, but the sharp cut-off by synaptic inhibition prevents the convergence of lagging, noisy spike inputs into a multiple-letter mix. The next synapses, in larger RFs with overlapping boundaries, temporally correlate the meaning of word groups into the context of the whole sentence, and so on with adjacent sentences. These temporal correlations of letters within words within sentences are separate due to the correlation of RF size with neural distance/latency, enforced by rapidly reemitting synapses, so that quick temporal correlations of letters are in small RFs, while the context of whole sentences has a longer latency that adds meaning in larger RFs. As with letters that make up words, the rapid inhibitory cutoff of slow spikes at serial synapses prevents sequential disorder of successive feature meanings from mixing at the same time in the same RF. Spatial and temporal summation of spikes reemitted from image sen-

---

[257] Words are identified within 90 msec, during reading fixations of more than 300 msec; in Ashby, J. & Kingston, J. (2009) Biol. Psychol. 80:84 and Hauk, O., Davis, M., Ford, M. (2006) Neuroimage 30:1383.

tences, create a context at a longer latency and neural distance from serially summated meanings.

Sustained spikes with fixed emission times maintain a constant distance/latency ratio in labeled lines; but this is not a latency code of letters to construct sentences centrally. Tremor during fixation synchronizes 2D spike emission from variable spatial and temporal input patterns; synchronized reemission of z spikes occurs at convergent synaptic stages of temporal and spatial integration as RF areas increase in size. The turnover of viewed words with each fixational transition, as emitted spikes at fixed times, continuously alters the reemitted context at the last integrative stage. This hierarchy of timed synchronies at serially convergent synapses reduces spike rates, which correlates with an increased latency of perceptual context at the distal, largest RFs. Spike emitted-times, mediated by single spikes or short spike bursts, also do not have information to rebuild images in distal RFs (*Fig. 4.1*).

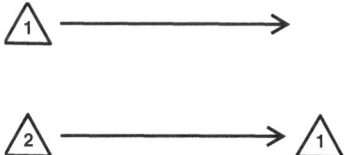

Fig. 4.1: Shown is that a z spike moves time as well as location. The spike '1' above, emits due to an edge event; the event time is fixed once the spike moves from the emitted location. The moved '1' in the lower figure has greater latency and distance magnitudes, coupled in a constant ratio, but still has the same '1' emitted time, as a 'micro-memory'. The new spike '2' in the same neuron has a serial emitted time sustained here by the presence of the same edge. The temporal synchrony of proximally sustained spikes at serial retinotopically aligned synapses, retains the fixed micro-memory time distally if rapidly reemitted. That RGC-synchronized spikes emitted at serial times phase-lock with distal z spikes, is facilitated by fixed axonal distances with repeatable spike latencies.

The durations of retinal slow potentials, the perceptual moment, minimal fixation period, and spike latencies to large IT RFs, are similar to the minimal latency of 150 msec after stimulus initiation, necessary to phase-lock disparate area rhythms over the whole visual cortex.[258] This figure is also close to the reading latencies of 150-170 msec in V4 and 180-200 msec in VWFA described by Dehaene (op. cit.). Spikes generated by newly read letters and words, retain a foveal resolution due to small cone RFs; during fixation, these peripheral spikes temporally append continuously, synchronizing with spikes that have lasted through successive convergent summations. The summed synaptic reemissions from distally latent spikes create a context and an increased cognitive analysis of the retinal information, which is not multiplexed or transmitted as information, but are reemitted spike times from successive synaptic filtering layers. This filtering distills an increasingly accurate context, or meaning, of the fixationally synchronized spikes, via distal spikes.[259]

Sequential reading saccades create a continuity, repeatedly attaching spikes into cortical reverberations lasting 500 msec, to bridge the shorter fixation peri-

---

[258] Roland, P., op. cit. Chap. Three, shows that spikes traverse cortical visual areas, from V1 to IT with different latencies, which loop back from later areas onto earlier areas to rapidly phase-lock these areas. Roland presents evidence that perception of apparent motion, of the same object presented twice with a spatial and temporal gap, results from integrative processes in V5 that synchronize over time with V1.

[259] As discussed at the end of the last chapter, successive summations can create a larger context and refined analysis of the same peripheral information. The increase in synapses in larger RFs can be interpreted as pooled inputs that probabilistically vote for behavioral choices (Britten, K., Newsom, W., Shadlen, M., Celebrini, S., Movshon, J. (1996) Vis. Neurosci. 13:87). Over time, behaviorally induced synaptic learning of logical decisions dominates instinctive fight-or-flight responses. Here, learned logic persists as altered synapses that facilitate repeated passage of synchronized fixed-memory z spikes.

ods; a temporally isolated word stimulus can create a crescendo of spike activity in cortex that peaks at five seconds.[260] This synchronized assembly line correlates the new spike initiation times, in a stream of retinal spikes, via stages of convergent z spike reemissions, which gain context from previous words and sentences. When input spikes do not converge on synapses with the correlated timing necessary to emit new spikes, the continuous impedance match of perception with new inputs may decouple, if the gap is hundreds of msec. The complexity of information is in the edges that stimulate high RGC rates; resulting convergent spike emissions enable accumulative, but delayed contexts to correlate with retinal informational complexity. Z spikes that reemit during several fixations, may integrate fixed memory-times at distal synapses, as new ideas in the stream of consciousness.

Why does zero phase lag in spikes temporally correlated over neural distances seem to violate the rules of causality? If one takes a simultaneous z section at any instant (*Fig. 4.2*), one finds enduring spikes at the distal cortex, and new spikes at the retina; this sequential order does not violate causality. If something abruptly changes in a complex environment, a cortical delay of hundreds of milliseconds is required to detect, perceive, analyze and organize an appropriate motor reaction, such as pressing a brake pedal;[261] unless subcortical reflexes subconsciously respond quickly to the coiled position of a rattlesnake or the looming baseball described in Chapter Three. This cortical delay to abrupt stimu-

---

[260] Dehaene, op. cit.

[261] Dashi, A., Tran, C., Wilder, M., Mazer, C., Trivedi, M. (2012) Cogn. Sci. 36:948.

lation into a later perceptual moment, also does not violate causality. That a perceptual moment has both cortical delay and new input, can be better understood by diagraming time on two axes below:

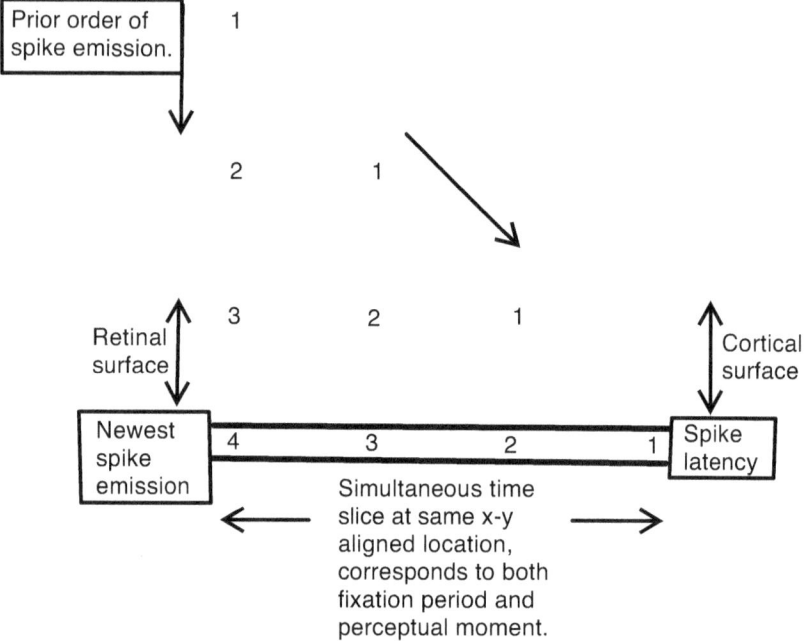

Fig. 4.2: This diagram synthesizes the two previous figures, showing one in a series of slices, or z sections, between the retinal surface and distal stages of cortex. The axes are 2D time linked to 2D anatomical locations on this 2D page. The z section shows a spike sequence of 4-3-2-1 in the perceptual moment, from a single edge, via the fastest neural route. If a fixation lasts 150 msec, this synchronizes a sequence of spikes in a perceptual moment lasting about the same 150 msec. A z spike "remembers" its emission time, quantified by the number in the diagram, if it reemits rapidly at synapses. Spike emitted times at constant speed have sequential distance/latency, shown by following the fixed '1' time diagonally. FEMs sustain spikes from layers of RGCs, which converge into the z section diagrammed, while transiently x-y aligned. New spikes are synchronously aligned with latent spikes; this process continues the perceptual moment. During fixation, x-y resolution does not smear into adjacent z sections, due to predominantly temporal convergence of spikes at LGN and V1 P cell levels, which retinotopically reiterate foveal resolution (see Fig. 3.3).

The curved retina receives simultaneous input at any instant of time; FEMs stimulate cyclical, x-y synchronized spikes from layers of RGCs. Subsequent surfaces reiterate retinotopy; as shown by Wedeen et al. (op. cit., Chap. One), these remain unitary x-y surfaces because they are not wired as a 3D spatial structure. Geometrically, the 2D surfaces are orthogonal to the moving 1D z spike locations. What is perceived externally as 3D spatial anatomy, is due to 3D perceptions that temporally summate from fixational spike synchronies at binocular synapses in retinotopic 2D arrays. Repeated retinotopic 2D surfaces reemit identical 1D z spikes, which are moving repetitious locations that converge at serial synapses, from the simultaneous x-y times of orthogonal, FEM-stimulated edges, emitted as RGC fixed times. Adjusting spike rates and speed, neural circuits have evolved to make LGN, V1 and subsequent arrays, phase-locked in time at serial synapses that facilitate the reemission of temporally synchronous input spikes. The transient positioning of sustained z spikes on converging z axes, makes static in time, the serial z spike synchronies induced by shifting of foveal RFs across image edges.

Here, spikes move fixed emission times as z locations across 2D surfaces, not coded x-y information. If new, sustained spikes are in the same elongated perceptual moment, they add fixed emission times, or additional peripheral detail as micro-memories that increase contextual perception of the same feature edge pattern. At 100 Hz, any z section in *Fig. 4.2* will have several z spikes, each with a fixed emission time, in temporally synchronous perception; this is similar to several musical notes heard at the same time and perceived as harmony.[262]

---

[262] Benade, A. (1992) <u>Horns, Strings and Harmony</u>.

Z equivalence may be necessary to explain how identical spikes, without novel encoded data, can synchronize, or phase-lock repeatedly, at convergent synapses. Labeled receptor types selectively respond to the complexity of peripheral features; sustained responses are fixed emission times that persist perceptually during fixation. In *Fig. 4.2*, these delayed RGC spikes attach to previously emitted z spikes in late-stage cortex, to become the continuity that comprises the perceptual moment. Also, RGC spikes sustained by image edges, rather than conveying data as a code over time, fix emission times by rapid reemission, which synchronize latently in distal RFs as convergent context.[263] If a cone RF boundary does not cross an image edge within a z section window, no spike emits to also z synchronize in the cortically linked, convergent RF. It is the synchronization of an edge-generated spike in the same z section (otherwise defined as a perceptual moment), with a cortical z spike that fixes the edge-timing as a perceived micro-memory.

We return to the flash-lag effect because the components of time diagrammed in *Fig. 4.2* make the simultaneous perception of a stationary flash and an advancing stimulus motion understandable without invoking an illusory 'prediction'. In this version of flash-lag, the flash and the adjacent motion stimuli initiate at the same time.[264] Cortical perception to both stimuli are delayed; the flash is perceived as static in spatial location over time, but the perception of stimulus motion is in real time because contrasty new RGC spike emitted times, due to ana-

---

[263] Sugase et al., op. cit., Chap. Three; sustained RGC responses have delayed emitted time micro-memories that summate later in IT cortex.

[264] Shimojo, S. (2014) Front. Psych. 5:196; version II is used here.

tomical division of labor, are sustained to precisely align with enduring, identical cortical z spikes with no x-y tags. Just as previously, the moving stimulus is perceived to move location over the same fixation period and z section that the flash is seen statically.

Other experiments are also explained by the simultaneous z section. Pursuit and identification of multiple visual targets integrate psychophysically as a single motion signal in the same perceptual moment,[265] best explained by multiple responses to different targets at separate M RGC locations that all synchronize with latent spikes in V5 cortex, a division of labor between RGCs and V5 that does not anatomically conflict. Conflict in the synchronous perceptual moment would occur if all targets transmitted time-multiplexed data to a cortical location.

Division of labor is also shown by cells in somatosensory cortex, which perceive the convergent spikes emitted by several types of skin receptors that respond separately to shape (SA), skin slip or speed (RA) and texture (PAC), but collectively reduce firing rates and increase RF areas successively in areas 3b, 1 and 2.[266] Similar to the response of visual cortex to flicker stimuli described in Chapter One, phase-locked entrainment of cell populations reduces in the successive areas in response to stimuli that range from 50 to 800 Hz. 4% of Area 3b cells, but no measurable Area 2 cells, synchronize when PAC receptors are stimulated at a maximal rate of 800 Hz, which is just perceptible.[267] If one

---

[265] Jin, Z., Watamaniuk, S., Potapchuk, E., Heinen, S. (2014) J. Neurosci. 34: 5835.

[266] Fisher, G., Freeman, B., Rowe, M. (1983) J. Neurophys. 49:75.

[267] Harvey, M., Saal, H., Dammann, J., Bensmaia, S. (2013) PLoS Biol. 11:e1001558.

texture vibration at low stimulus intensity induces one PAC spike,[268] this frequency does not have to be transmitted to the same cortical cell for 800 spikes/sec to be perceived. Extending the univariance of Li et al. in Chapter One to cortical cells, neurons that fire to convergent synchronous inputs within the larger x-y aligned 3b (or Area 1) RF can skip firing, or trade off as adaptation occurs; the cortically pooled phase-locking occurs at lower frequency in any specific cell. According to Harvey et al., the ability to discriminate frequencies perceptually in humans, correlates with the collective phase-locked and intensity responses to the same stimulatory frequencies measured in monkey somatosensory cells. Individual cell and pooled cell spike rates, which phase-lock, correlate highest in time in cells of Area 3b. Increased spike rate, a response to stimulus intensity, and phase-locking, a response to stimulus frequency, occur in the same cells. The fact that they increase together in the same cells indicates a causal relationship; that is, higher instantaneous rates of, here, identical spikes, are necessary to convergently synchronize at some cells (this specificity may adapt by moving to other cells and times in the same cortical RF). This induces a stronger and quicker phase-locked response, which in *Fig. 4.2* is required for delayed distal perceptions of sensory labeled spike frequency responses.

Fine stimulus texture that induces high PAC spike rates confounds with a course texture at higher slip speed, which both induce the same spike rate in many cells in Areas 3b, 1 and 2. However, cells in Areas 1 and 2 also display texture-only responses or speed-only responses, indicating inhibitory convergence that subtracts and separates RA and PAC la-

---

[268] Bensmaia, S. (2008) Behav. Brain Res. 190:165.

beled inputs.[269] If RA is subtracted, an invariant percept of fine texture results despite varying scan speeds at the skin. Here, rather than multiplexed information, identical spikes in labeled receptors retain the emitted times at the sensory surface in the convergent cortical circuit. That speed or texture is perceived depends on timely circuit output spikes in the RA or PAC labeled neuron in cortical areas, which synchronize with their respective sensory receptor labels in the aligned RF. Edge vibrations cause PAC spike frequencies with a precision and a detectability of less than a msec.[270] Area 1 and 2 z spikes that periodically reemit from synchronous 3b inputs correlate a latent cortical percept of sensory stability, with peripheral spikes of the same label.

The convergence of SA, RA and PAC labeled neurons at the same cortical synapse, reemits unlabeled spikes into long-latency perception; the cortical preservation of labeled sustained and phase-locked responses in the same group of cells is conventionally called multiplexing of information over time. However, here z spikes do not move information, but permit anatomical division of labor between precise labeled receptor responses and convergent delayed perceptions, at the same time in the same x-y aligned RF, as shown in *Fig. 4.2*. Precise labeled perceptions result if *any* convergent identical z spike in any neuron in the aligned cortical RF periodically reemits and is synchronous with any PAC repetitive spikes. That sustained rates and phase-locked responses colocate in the same cortical neurons may result because increased stimulus intensity recruits

---

[269] Depeault, A., Meftah, el-M., Chapman, C. (2013) J. Neurophys. 110:1554.

[270] Mackevicius, E., Best, M., Saal, H., Bensmaia, S. (2012) J. Neurosci. 32:15309.

additional input into the mean cortical spike rates, which increase the convergent phase-locking of a pooled response. Because various sensory neuron types fire spikes in the same z section as older re-emitted cortical z spikes, the percept of fixed time in the older, unlabeled z spike, if reemitted at multiple synapses, loses precise stimulus timing, but still synchronizes during fixation with newly generated, RF-aligned spike times as diagrammed in *Fig. 4.2*. Precise new spikes at a sensory RF temporally synchronize with reemitted distal spikes if sustained gamma rhythms are measured to phase-lock with population-averaged cortical slow theta rhythms.[271]

The sensory hierarchy of spatially and temporally convergent spikes that reemit to higher areas only when inputs synchronize, has the same proportionality of neural distance/latency, that spatially separates, at the same synchronous time, levels of perceptual integration, as stated earlier for reading. Distally latent spikes that summate from rapid receptor shifting (*Fig. 3.3*) or from texture PAC inputs (above), impedance match with the same area/time ratio, the large temporal and spatial dimensions of aligned cortical RFs, to confer a synchronous z stability on the rapid, jittery x-y timing of small peripheral sensory RFs. Synaptically filtered, older cortical z spikes are fewer,[272] distributed over larger numbers of neurons, at slower rates and slower average frequencies in larger cell populations in larger perceptual RFs; these phase-lock with RF-aligned, sustained identical spikes in labeled peripheral neurons. A z section impedance matches a maintained spike

---

[271] Panzeri, S., Ince, R., Diamond, M., Kayser, C. (2014) Philos. Trans. R. Soc. B Biol. Sci. 369: 20120467.

[272] Wolfe, J., Houwelling, A., Brecht, M. (2010) Curr. Opin. Neurobio. 20:306; Barth, A. & Poulet, J. (2012) Trends Neurosci. 35:345.

movement with the proportional distance/latency of increasing RF areas from retina to IT cortex (*Fig. 5*). Spike rate and speed (distance/time) correlate at each synaptic stage, to reduce spike rate and increase spike interval to more distant and larger RFs. Fixationally sustained emitted spike times synchronize serial stages at each sequential fixed instant. Additionally, sustained fixed-time spikes reverberate among cells as short-term or working memory.

With memory, one can stop the transition of time from a recent event, thus preventing the sensation of an event from consciously expiring, by recurrently exciting neural firing in networks of neurons.[273] Persistent spiking is a general phenomenon with short-term memory,[274] but the experimental paradigm, in which the animal waits attentively for a stimulus in order to use what it has learned, confounds a historical memory, as temporally equivalent to a future (predictive) plan.[275]

Does sustained firing from new events nullify the previous sustained spikes that now persist as short-term memory? When spikes move at fixed speeds in neurons, their fixed emission times (*Fig. 4.1*) synchronously and quickly summate at synapses, to retain emission times as a persistent recurrent memory. Similar to the times fixed by frames in a film, recurrent z spikes make the fixed times of a visual

---

[273] Fuster, J. (2001) Neuron 30:319; first gave evidence that sustained neuronal firing also sustains recent, or working memory.

[274] Major & Tank, (2004), op. cit. Chap. Three.

[275] Curtis, C. & Conolly, J. (2008) J. Neurophys. 99:133; the nature of time as location, in backward memory and with forward imagination, stated in Chap. Two, applies also to future planning. 'Prospective' future-looking cells are intermingled among working memory cells; in Quintana, J. & Fuster, J. (1999) Cereb. Cortex 9:213.

image persist as a short-term memory, without an explicit code of image information.[276] Sustained firing may exist in either sensory or memory types of neurons, but its effect is defined by the neuron's direct connection to a sensory receptor or indirect coupling to conscious sensation by spiking synchronies. Because image data is not encoded, fixed spike times (micro-memories) of working memory in prefrontal cortex[277] do not anatomically or perceptually conflict with the continuous temporal gamma synchronization of retinotopically mapped z spikes between retina and V1 cortex.[278]

So rather than spikes with image data that traverse distance to an addressed location where the memory is cortically encoded, spikes with a constant speed, phase-lock rapidly at specific cortical distances synchronously timed with fixed spike emission times. Long-term memory retrieval can be defined as the activation of a spatial location in cortex via the hippocampus, a location modified at the original historical event. Reactivation of this synaptically facilitated location, creates a sense of the time of the original event, and thus of the event, without decoding over time the peripheral information that initiated the spikes. Because time always accompanies distance, no matter its mapped direction, fixed emission times (as micro-memories) are at different synaptic distances. It is known that with development from age seven to adulthood, the fusiform face area, which is a part of IT cortex devoted

---

[276] Rolls & Tovee, op. cit. Chap. Three.

[277] Fuster, J. (2008) The Prefrontal Cortex.

[278] Z spike micro-memories may explain this lack of conflict, as posed in Bettencourt, K. & Xu Y. (2016) Nature Neurosci. 19:150; here, z axis spikes are a moving location/time dimension orthogonal to the V1 x-y synaptic layers that reemit as short term memory-times.

to the recognition of faces, increases area several times. The parahippocampal place area that recognizes places, also increases in area.[279] These increases are correlated with better memory for faces and places, and likely are due to greater stimulation and volume of recurrent spikes synchronously re-emitted from more synapses.

Upon memory retrieval, phase-locking of spikes in hippocampal, parahippocampal and medio-temporal cortical locations is observed.[280] Time, or memory, phase-locks spikes in hippocampal and neocortical areas into synchrony, to temporarily and temporally bind as a single z location. The hippocampus is organized as a memory-as-location spatial map that is prominently developed in rodents. The increase in cortical topography in humans has to result from greater memory quantities over a longer, stimulus-rich lifespan, and so is more than a neuronal simulacrum of environmental topography. A memory may not be "stored", like a bit of information in computer memory, but sequential events may be associated as adjacent synaptic locations that transpose distance for time, synchronizing with the fixed emission times of reverberating z spikes.

If memory recall was not defined by 2D surface location, could gene mutations code for an infinity of instantly recalled images? Does this recalled imagery replicate the spike timing of the original event? There is no doubt that generic biochemical activity facilitates transmissibility at synapses, and

---

[279] Golari, G., Ghahremani, D., Whitfield-Gabrieli, S., Reiss, A., Eberhardt, J., Gabrieli, J., Grill-Spector, K. (2007) Nature Neurosci. 10:512.

[280] Axmacher, N., Mormann,F., Fernandez, G., Fell, J. (2006) Brain Res. Rev. 52:170; Csicsuari et al., op. cit.

that dendritic spines expand for short-term and long-term learning and memory.[281] It is this activation of a specific location, as an enlarged dendritic spine, which constitutes the equivalence here of location as a fixed time and memory. Dendritic spines form and dissolve[282] in large quantities at microscopic levels. A memory engram is defined as a discrete group of neurons that form lasting synaptic and dendritic changes to a sensory event. However, a true memory is not readily distinguishable from a false memory that is artificially induced in hippocampal cells in a context unrelated to the original sensory event. Both true and false memories overlap in the same cells and have the same increase in general gene activity. The complex neural connections induced by memories use large regions of evolutionarily conserved genes that activate as a set, rather than DNA that mutates over time to adapt.[283] Similar memories with common elements, do have different spike intervals that correlate with differing trial delays and other experimental conditions.[284]

Local neural circuits have similar gamma frequencies despite organism size, but transiently phase-lock with rhythms that do not scale, but depend on hippocampal size. In humans this hippocampal rhythm

---

[281] Li, F. & Tsien, J. (2009) New Engl. J. Med. 361:13; Hempel, C., Hartman, K., Wang, X., Turrigiano, G., Nelson, S. (2000) J. Neurophys. 83:3031; Hill, T. & Zito, K. (2013) J. Neurosci. 33:678.

[282] If one examines dendritic or spike morphology at high resolution, an increase in information is found; see Butts et al., op. cit. Chap. Three. Similar is the increase in fractal length with magnification.

[283] Ramirez, S., Tonegawa, S., Liu, X. (2013) Front. Behav. Neurosci. 7:226; Liscovitch-Brauer, N., Alon, S., Porath, H., Elstein, B., Unger, R., Ziv, T., Admon, A., Levanon, E., Rosenthal, J., Eisenberg, E. (2017) Cell 169:191. Complex behaviors require complex gene activities but do not require genetic mutations to encode the behavior.

[284] Eichenbaum, H. (2014) Nature Rev. Neurosci. 15:732.

is in the delta band, 1-4 Hz. In carnivores this band is at 4-6 Hz, and in rodents, this hippocampal rhythm is in the theta band, at 4-11 Hz.[285] With this distance/frequency proportionality, phase-locking occurs at a specific location, but is slightly out of phase in adjoining areas recorded at the same time nearby. Assuming a constant spike speed, here these phase differences do not store data but indicate that synchronization at the same or similar frequencies occurs at nearby locations of synapses. Synchronization associates memories, as fixed emitted times, with cortical locations of contiguous memory-modified synapses.

Spike synchronization of memory recall at distinct cortical locations is similar to the synchronization of perceptual maps in several cortical areas in the binding problem. As postulated by von der Malsberg, the various perceptual attributes attached to an object require a temporal correlation, within 1-10 msec, of spikes in a few or many neurons, in separate neural locations.[286] He raises several questions: different spatial correlations are required to differentiate the perceptual pattern due to one object from that due to another; the synchrony due to one object also has to be temporally differentiated from that due to another. In addition, the temporal code for a specific visual image cannot vary or confound with other visual stimuli. Moreover, a synchronization over time, of two spikes separated by any distance, can be coincidental neural interactions that do not necessarily bind stimuli and their quali-

---

[285] Buzsaki et al., op. cit. Chap. One; Jacobs, J., Kahana, M., Ekstrom, A., Fried, I. (2007) J. Neurosci. 27:3839.

[286] Von der Malsberg, C. (1999) Neuron 24:95; Singer, W., Engel, A., Kreiter, A., Munk, M., Neuenschwander, S., Roelfesema, P. (1997) Trends Cogn. Sci. 1:252, analyze synchrony as a binding mechanism.

ties. Ergo, here it follows that for synchrony to be a mechanism for perceptual binding, spikes cannot store or code image information. As explained here, dynamic information temporally coded in spikes would conflict if synchronously timed at aligned, distant RFs. This information would otherwise become static during fixation, when spikes synchronize over time. But if spikes as visualized here, are fixed emission times that always move, they can continuously adapt z latencies of synchronous, FEM generated z times at various cortical perceptual locations as dynamic retinal information changes.

Researchers have attempted to analyze how features 'bind' into perceived objects via experiments that show 'illusory conjunctions'.[287] For example, the misperception of one object's color or shape with that of another object may be due to a short stimulus presentation time. Other misperceptions occur due to apposition of distractors or the creative disruption of expected conjunctions. Letters in a word may be perceptually misplaced with letters in an adjacent word under certain conditions. If the location of the object is not purposely obfuscated, the conjunction of location and its features increase the probability of the correct perception. But some experiments show that proximal 'preattentive' processes have more illusory conjunctions than distal latent cognitive processes. Labeled receptor RFs have specific locations on the retina, so the increased probability that the retinal location and the feature at that location are perceptually bound is a proximal process. Here, this conjunctive identity is due to division of labor, in that features are not spike-encoded to be sent to a distal perceptual location as multiplexed information, but are synchronous, at the

---

[287] Wolfe, J. & Cave, K. (1999) Neuron 24:11.

same time, as the latent perception as shown in *Fig. 4.2*. The fact that here, identical z spikes are required for synchrony and do not code image features, allows, under experimental conditions, an abnormal illusory conflict due to juxtaposition of those features. Binding does not have different distal population codes for differing object features;[288] here endurance of z spikes in time and space synchronizes at each instant, with x-y aligned proximally differentiated retinal information.

Labeled inputs to specific retinotopic maps, must overlap at the same time under synchronized firing conditions, so that the percepts labeled separately for color, movement, shape, etc. bind because the same 2D location phase-locks on all the maps. An object, at the same x-y position in the image and on repeated retinotopic maps, has its various qualities bind because aligned z spikes transit parallel x-y locations. A memory is also not confused with other memories, due to consistent mapping to a distinct location on all 2D surfaces.[289] A large part of neural noise, must be 'searches' of spike fixed emission times in short-term memory that try to match the distance/time marking a long-term memory's cortical surface location. While subliminal searches may not be perceived, synchrony is, due to increased duration and quantity of z spikes recurring between distributed maps over time. The view here is, z spike emitted times repeatedly activate synapses at a distinct location, previously modified by conserved

---

[288] Gray, C. (1999) Neuron 24:31; Singer, W. (1999) Neuron 24:49,

[289] Memory as a specific x-y location can be resilient to cortical ablation, due to remapping by equivalent topographical z inputs from other areas to the remaining cortical area; this makes the anatomically diffuse memory code of Hebb, D. (1949) The Organization of Behavior, logically compatible with synchronous z spikes at x-y maps.

genes and their factors, at a distance/time correlated with the time of memory origin, rather than instantly retrieving stored genetic mutations that encode the data comprising the distinct memory.

The problem of perceptual binding shows that conscious time depends on circuit components made simultaneous in time, by the passage of multiple identical z spikes at an objective instant in time, between two disparate neural locations. If the concept of 'time' is a perception dependent on spatial properties, such as that existing between macro-space and the retina's surface, we should disambiguate it. For example, we have a time comprised of 'doing time', that is occupying space with no movement or activity, except for temporal aging. We also have time that is directly proportional to distance traversed, which gives us a constant speed, like the speed of light. As already noted, time is measured with atomic accuracy, at millions of cycles per second, and also in cycles of months for sidereal time. Time is sequential, as conventionally used, yet also acts simultaneously, on multiple parallel inputs, at temporally convergent synapses.

Fig. 4.2 shows that 2D time can accentuate the msec precision of an x-y edge moving across the retinal plane, so is not a convergent blurring of the cortical perceptual moment, which persists for 150 msec on the z axis. A static spike cannot store memory, but synchronous spike emissions that correlate with the fixed times of retinal edge-crossings can retain the timing of image stimulation at distal locations without transmitting a code to reconstuct the image. That time has multiple components separable when plotted as shown in *Fig. 4.2*, has been unexplored till now, because generic time is still more useful in science as a single standard.

In computer systems, the synthesis of information from various sensors with microcontrollers and display devices requires temporal synchronization and calibration, due to differences in gain, clock and sample rates of the connected instruments.[290] Yet physiologically, such internal inconsistencies are filtered out, because a regulatory master clock is replaced in brains by sustained spikes from receptors that converge at synapses in serial 2D surfaces, which reemit output spikes into perceptual awareness only if input spikes are spatially and temporally synchronous. Here, the z spikes do not encode or decode image information; but peripheral responses synchronize with latent cortical spikes during fixation, over neural z distance (*Fig. 4.2*). Rather than an internal clock that requires a precise and expensive calibration of components, moving spikes have emitted-times (*Fig. 4.1*) from image edge crossings, not a latency code, which synchronize in least-time at RF-aligned convergent synapses. Perception of precision is due to proximal sustained spikes that are synchronous at any instant with distal cortical spikes in an aligned RF.[291] The synchronized, re-emitted frequency is inversely proportional to neural distance/spike latency between linked synapses.[292]

---

[290] In Lin, S.-S. & Bajcsy, R. (2006) J. Opt. Soc. Amer. A **23**:2997.

[291] Montemurro, M., Rasch, M., Murayama, Y., Logothetis, N., Panzeri, S. ((2008) Curr. Biol. **18**:375; as just discussed, sustained rates colocate with synchrony in the same somatosensory cells. Spike rate/sec in one cell scales to pooled synchrony averaged over many cells.

[292] *Fig. 3.3* shows that tremor movement in the x-y plane, and z spike movement, provide the two dimensions of time plotted in *Fig. 4.2*. The orthogonal axes show that spike latency from the retina to the cortex may not sync with the fixed emission time of that spike; this affects where least-time reemission occurs. This is true also of photonic least-time; a mirage, caused by hot air at a large surface, creates a longer but faster light route, which impinges with straight light synchronously in time at the retinal surface. A 2D time plot visualizes the synchronously timed perceptual moments that include a mirage.

The fixed times of spikes sustained by an object edge at an RGC RF, allows a stable percept of object location and timing, as *Figs. 3.3 and 4.2* show.

One must discuss here the reliable and precise latencies from stimulated rodent whiskers. If a single whisker is stimulated, due to topographic identity, an electrode in the corresponding cortically aligned RF records the first spike with a least-time latency, reliable over many trials. The fastest spike identifies the nearest whisker that stimulated the cortical cell.[293] Following spikes and nearby whiskers with afferents that converge on the same barrel column, have variably delayed spike latencies. But the convergence of initial spikes in multiple fibers with the same least-time latency synchronizes cells in the barrel column, which quickly reemit spikes from the stimulated whisker. The event-emitted spike times that synchronize at a convergent synapse fix micro-memories that are retained as the spike moves distally (*Fig. 4.1*). As spike distance/latency is a constant ratio or speed proximally-distally, rapidly re-emitted spike times are stable references that synchronize emitted with reemitted spikes. Spike micro-memories phase-lock at the same RF-aligned synapses in serial arrays, if sustained from the same receptor RF and image edge as previous, now distal spikes. As already described for the perceptual moment in Chapter Three, sustained spikes may emit later but are not 'older', they are new micro-memories that attach to previously emitted z spikes now in distal cortex. Newly sustained proximal spikes temporally synchronize sensory data with now latent, fixed-times of cortical z percept-spikes.

---

[293] Panzeri et al., op. cit.; described is a tactile 2D surface version of experiments referenced in Chap. Three, in which visually stimulated spikes converge on an RGC via the shortest least-time route.

If identical spikes spatially and temporally synchronize at synapses, emitted fixed times reemit as micro-memories that synchronize at each convergent synapse. In computer graphics, it is necessary to stitch together 2D mats into a continuous surface without overlaps or gaps. Algorithmic round-off errors that accumulate over distance have required jury-rigged solutions to reconnect the 2D mats continuously. A similar problem occurs when a camera pans horizontally; the successive frames may not transition smoothly and rapidly if the large amount of repeated image information is not reduced to allow integration within the duration of the perceptual moment. External holograms use previously calibrated and synchronized laser light to create externally perceived 3D structures. In physiological vision, temporally and spatially asynchronous light inputs upon the dual retinas become a single image, via tremor-timed synchrony of spikes converging at binocular synapses that reemit.   These examples synchronize emitted-reemitted z spikes, which retain memory times without distally decoded information.

Another relevant sensory phenomenon is the lack of perception of the optic disc region of the retina; convergent cortical areas simply ignore the optic disc, with no emitted z spikes with no initial x-y locations. Neural mechanisms have no difficulty with the tasks of the last paragraph because FEM-gated spikes sustain during fixation; RGC emitted spikes reemit to endure into perception, which synchronize with new RGC edge crossings. Rather than externally imposed x-y coordinates, temporal and spatial convergence at synapses, such as in oriented V1 RFs, filters out mistimed spikes by rapidly reemitting synchronously timed inputs. Retinal RF-aligned spikes transmit no x-y labeled data or coordinates, but only z location and time, which synchronize latent distal perception with proximal sensory data.

Read & Cumming (op. cit. Chapter One) show that monocular images match as a stereo image via x-y aligned temporal summation at specific binocular V1/V2 synapses. Unbroken external image lines become perceptual via the FEM synchronized fixed emission times of RGC spikes, which converge at simple cells to rapidly reemit a retinal memory of an unbroken line. If retinal imagery is conventionally encoded as bits, the information digitizes upon transforming graded plexiform potentials to RGC spikes. Likewise, an externally broken line could be accidentally transmitted as a continuous line at a spatially convergent synapse, if image information was transmitted and decoded over time. But least-time light rays at image edges are a stable reference that impedance matches with contrasty spike responses. To repeat, FEM-gated emitted time is intrinsic to the moving locations of identical spikes at constant speed, which synchronously converge at univariant synapses; these quickly reemit, to z synchronize proximal RGC and distal IT, without moving x-y information. Variable delayed spikes sustained during the fixation period synchronize as a gist or added contextual detail. Because a neuron's 1D z spikes are here, not multiplexing multi-dimensional information, convergent distal perceptions latently synchronize with aligned image edges (*Fig. 4.2*) via spikes emitted at shifty RGC RF boundaries. Repeated retinotopy, coupled with precise spike timing at convergent synapses, reemits z spikes that are synchronously perceived due to inhibition of laggard spikes at the synapse. This enduring z continuity is not cortically static or decoded from a retinal code summed over time, but a transient, mobile process.

It is useful to compare the z section scheme in *Fig. 4.2* with current learning algorithms, which variously describe a comprehensive reduction of collective image dimensions (i.e. information), to few dimensions. Recognition of words or images via 'deep learning' couples convolutional neural networks with 'stochastic gradient descent',[294] in which serial layers of pluralistic neurons with many connections, refine an approximation from temporally coded data reiterated through a cyclical algorithm; concentrated computation over time pools an abstract output, learns a new pattern or converges on an identification of a previously learned template. This massive distributed computation while analogous, is not as good as brains, which have many synaptic connections in several cortical layers that quickly categorize and identify a stimulus in one passage or at most a few reverberations of stimulus-emitted spikes. The distally reemitted least-time synchrony of *Fig. 4.2*, uses the convergent 1D property of identical z spikes, not temporally coded data, to identify or abstract from words or images.

New chip design paradigms compress information into time-multiplexed spikes, while also requiring that temporally coded data moves to computational destinations. The information packets are time stamped and addressed to specialized units and distributed memory stores, which are routed around the central von Neumann bottleneck[295] (similar to spatial and temporal convergence at RGCs that

---

[294] LeCun, Y., Bengio, Y., Hinton, G. (2015) Nature 521:436.

[295] See Ganguli, S. & Sompolinsky, H. (2012) Ann. Rev. Neurosci. 35:485; Merolla, P., Arthur, J., Alvarez-Icaza, R., Cassidy, A., Sawada, J., Akopyan, F., Jackson, B., Imam, N., Guo, C., Nakamura, Y., Brezzo, B., Vo, I., Esser, S., Appuswamy, R., Taba, B., Amir, A., Flickner, M., Risk, W., Manohar, R., Modha, D. (2014) Science 453:668.

transmit spikes through the optic nerve). This contrasts with *Fig. 4.2* in which spikes are locations/emitted times that converge at synapses, to synchronize with but not encode external imagery, requiring no temporal code or decoding. Z spikes serially move constant distance/time ratios, which here, retain emitted times distally.

Physiologically, the sudden appearance of an image causes a higher rate of spikes impinging on convergent synapses in visual cortex, to cause a faster and more intense perception of the usually delayed stimulus percept, which by looming as it gets closer, increases the retinal area that then emits more spikes.[296] These temporally summate quickly to reduce reaction time so have an obvious protective function. A higher proximal spike rate has a high temporal resolution that is perceived if coupled, or synchronized, with distal z spikes in serially aligned RFs. Image stability and 3D stereo definition here are coupled in the same identical convergent z spikes, which requires gamma frequencies of monocular x-y spikes that reemit in z synchrony from convergent binocular cells. Also, spike rate alters time perceptions, shown in correlated increases in duration of spike rate induced with longer stimulus elapsed times, experimentally recorded in 'time' measuring cells in the hippocampal CA1 area.[297]

What is the primeval source of time? How does the sense of time evolve in neurons? A single action potential is transient and floating, unless another action potential occurs in the same linked neuron at

---

[296] Fotowat, H. & Gabbiani, F. (2007) J. Neurosci. 27:10047; the high spike rates found in locusts are analogous to the increased fractionation of time subjectively perceived by humans as an accident unfolds.

[297] Eichenbaum, op. cit.

the same time, as measured with an exogenous clock and multiple recording electrodes. These two transient APs are now comparable, since they occur at topographically identical neurons at the same measured time and in the same z section. Spikes naturally indicate sequence because they do not normally overtake one another. The mature neuron is immobile in space and time, in contrast to the proportional time and location of the spike. The frequency of moving z spikes, as locations/times in labeled neurons, synchronously reemits at reduced rate from convergent synapses at each serial x-y aligned surface. The transient positions of z spikes at synchronization frequencies impedance match with static RF-aligned arrays as one x-y-z entity.

Time responsive cells are interspersed with place cells in the hippocampus; Eichenbaum identifies the same cell as responsive to time and place, alternating in function; some neurons respond to time duration and spatial location at the same time. Cell response to elapsed time is independent of place, distance or motion of the stimulus, although some cells respond to multiple factors. The additive duration of firing in time cells, proportional to time elapsed, also is proportional to perceived distance to a serial landmark. Why is time duration interchangable with place memory in these cells? Moving spikes have time imbedded in fixed emission times; each spatial axis mapped in the hippocampus must also be coupled with time, as indicated in *Fig. 4.2*. That sustained spikes map, or locate an external place at a hippocampal synapse, means that repeated z spikes are necessary to modify the synapse, to reinforce a spatial location in the place cell. The quality of 'time' may be defined by 1D spike rates in individual time cells; synchronous orthogonal 1D spike convergence at a 2D location in a neuronal array may map x-y positions in the same cells as 'places'.

A similar set of experiments argues that time *is* memory, in heterogeneous spike patterns circulating as short-term memory in prefrontal cortex.[298] These spike patterns were found to differ with the specific trial delay period, even though the trial delay was not part of the memory task at hand. Using analytical techniques to separate out memory components, the investigators found that time composed more than 57% of the 6 factors found relevant to memory, and that time and memory are separate processes in large cell populations. But in the single neuron itself, time was the only factor experimentally relevant in the memory task. This corresponds with the concept here that the fixed emission time of a new spike is a micro-memory. One can conclude that averaging obscures the identification of simple mechanisms of memory formation.

The connections of place cells with hexagonal arrays of grid cells (GR) are still only somewhat defined.[299] GRs are located in the input-output area of the hippocampus, the medial entorhinal cortex (mEC) shown in *Fig. 2.2*. The mEC is positioned to control input to place cells, but laminar tracts from cortex also traverse the area.[300] However, place cells converge to GRs if the halved spike rates in GRs are a

---

[298] Machens, C., Romo, R., Brody, C. (2010) J. Neurosci. 30:350.

[299] Hafting, T., Fyhn, M., Molden, S., Moser, M., Moser, E. (2005) Nature 436:801.

[300] Kerr, K., Agster, K., Furtak, S., Burwell, R. (2007) Hippocampus 17:617; Witter, M., Naber, P., van Haaften, T., Machielsen, W., Rombouts, S., Barkhof, F., Sheltens, P., Lopes da Silva, F. (2000) Hippocampus 10:398; Bonnavie, T., Dunn, B., Fyhn, M., Hafting, T., Derdikman, D., Kubie, J., Roudi, Y., Moser, E., Moser M. (2013) Nature Neurosci. 16:309.

sign of convergence. Each place cell fires to a specific location in environmental space; GRs fire at the vertices of convergent hexagonal inputs so must cognitively connect locations as the animal moves by them. In keeping with this idea, spikes recorded at place cells and GRs precess in phase, or fire earlier in a cycle of the theta rhythm, as the distance to an external landmark looms closer. The precession is measured to be highest in single running trials, but averaging the data from many trials to reduce the variance in individual trials destroys this phase differential.[301] The measured theta phase shifts and maximal spike rates increase as a landmark becomes closer, which may jointly encode a map of spatial location; however, they are weakly correlated when graphed together, perhaps because spikes in individual cells do not fire at every cycle of the theta rhythm, which is averaged from cells near an electrode location.[302] Here, rather than a reconstructed map, spikes with precise fixed-times from external visual landmarks, synchronously converge at neurons, creating rapid gamma rhythms in several brain areas, while also augmenting the amplitude of a phase in the slow theta rhythm in the hippocampus.[303] An increase in frequency in the

---

[301] Reifenstein, E., Kempfer, R., Schreiber, S. Stemmler, M., Herz, A. (2012) PNAS (USA) 109:6301; the higher specificity of individual trials compared to pooled trials is discussed in the next chapter.

[302] Reifenstein, E., Stemmler, M., Herz, A., Kempfer, R., Schreiber, S. (2014) PLoS One 9:e100638; they also show that spikes measured at an elapsed time, are not statistically distinguishable from an elapsed distance, in single-run responses recorded at a place cell, in accord with the Eichenbaum data a few paragraphs back. This data also conforms with the statement that at constant spike speed (and path traversal speed), distance and time covary at local groups of cells.

[303] Lisman, J. (2005) Hippocampus 15:913 discusses gamma frequency integration at specific phases of the slower theta rhythm in hippocampus and cortex; also in Panzeri et al. op. cit.

theta band in some local cells as a landmark looms is interpreted as a phase advance compared with the nearby phase-locked frequencies averaged from many cells. This larger pool of spikes makes a local variance in synchronized wavelength seem like a phase shift. Cells in CA1 and CA3 areas show a 90-120 degree phase shift, due to the difference in the synchronized theta frequency or wavelength, between locations.[304] It is conventionally thought that phase differences in an averaged rhythm are transferred stores of information; here it is the local frequency synchronies, of arrayed cells at different distances, which correlate with the distances to looming landmarks at retinal receptors. In fact, desynchronization occurs with increased behavioral performance, indicating that local synchronies with varied wavelengths, usually lost in the averaged theta rhythm, are necessary to learn the detailed behavioral sequence.[305] Each external location may transiently phase-lock GR spike rate and an increasing contraction in theta wavelength as the distal looms closer at each serial landmark. This couples the retinal stimulation of spikes at sequential place cells to the spikes elicited from GRs, to synchronize landmark-stimulated RGC fixed emission times with hippocampal reemitted spikes.

For fixed spike times impinging on hippocampal synapses, reemission has to be rapid to retain the RGC micro-memories of image edges and synchronized hippocampal responses to the same, which is also necessary for veridical IT cortex categorization of

---

[304] Mizuseki, K., Sirota, A. Pastelkova, E., Buzsaki, G. (2009) Neuron 64:267.

[305] Mizuseki, K. & Buzsaki, G. (2013) Philos. Trans. R. Soc. Lond. B Biol. Sci. 369:20120530; synchrony occurs transiently at different locations, which is seen as desynchronization while learning a behavior.

sensory objects via synchronized spike emissions. Hippocampal interneuron synchronization has a precision of less than 1 msec, which is thought to be caused by equal neural distances from upstream PYCs and matched conduction delays, not due to adjacent gap junctions or contiguous dendritic arbors.[306] Here, this synchronous hippocampal state at a restricted set of x-y aligned synapses, quickly reemits z spikes in least-time in that z section, for a precise hippocampal phase lock onto the edges of each serially looming landmark.

When spikes phase-lock, as a hypothetical memory is recalled or a perception gels, the synchronized wavelength is determined by the distance and latency of spikes at specific synapses. But simultaneous APs are sequential in a neuron due to appearance, then disappearance (*Fig. 4.1*). That two locations sequence time is implicit in the design of clocks. A moving location, the pointer, rotates to discrete stationary locations marked sequentially on a dial. The simultaneous event, of the same pointer that moves past different dial markings, tells us that time moves sequentially in repeated synchrony.

Dancers perceive when their kick is precisely coordinated with their neighbors' even though there are 150 msec perceptual delays, various neuronal distances and differences in spike latencies throughout the sensory and motor systems. The knowledge of precise coordination exists, in the dancer and in observers, seemingly in real time, because our orthogonal retina emits spikes directly stimulated by the sequence of external events; z spikes are in x-y synchrony due to tremor-gating. A section in a mo-

---

[306] Diba, K., Amardsingham, A., Mizsuseki, K. Buzsaki, G. (2014) J. Neurosci. 34:14984; gamma rhythms also did not create precision.

tion sequence (*Fig. 4.2*) shows not only the high rate of sustained proximal emission times, but also displays converging synchronies that ascend in duration to the latent cortical percept. Each synchronized z section, due to juxtaposition with other z sections, adds into a causal, coordinated sequence.

The x-y-z accuracy of visuo-motor sequence is shown in flocks of 'roller' pigeons, with eyes laterally positioned so that 180 degree visual fields have a slight overlap in front of the bird. The horizontal area of the pigeon retina,[307] analogous to the primate fovea, x-y aligns with those of birds flying nearby. Flocking pigeons are, in effect, a multiple-organism version of the repeated retinotopic maps in a primate's visual system. APs sustained from midget RGCs, as shown in the last chapter, emit in synchronous tremor-gated unison as stimulus edges cross foveal RF edges, to converge on V1 simple cells. A flock of pigeons, composed of a repeated overlap of visual fields, synchronizes APs throughout the 2D surfaces of parallel visual systems, so reacts subliminally with short latencies in the optic tectum (a pigeon's evolutionarily earlier version of the SC)[308] to create the highly coordinated sweeps and curves of flocking behavior. This rapid response occurs because orthogonal z APs reemit from retinotopically aligned surfaces in least-time (*Fig. 3.3*).[309]

---

[307] Hayes, B., Hodos, W., Holden, A., Low, J. (1987) Vis. Res. 27:31

[308] The optic tectum is a much larger part of brain volume in fish and birds compared to the SC in mammals (Wikipedia, anonymous entry).

[309] The dependence of aggregate flocking behavior on spatial x-y location, but independent of distance among adjacent birds, is in Ballerini, M., Cabibbo, N., Candelier, R., Cavagna, A., Cisbani, E., Giardina, I., Leconte, V., Orlandi, A., Parisi, G., Procaccini, A., Viale, M., Zdravkovic, V. (2008) PNAS (USA) 105:1232. This rapidly reactive flocking structure is analogous to the z distance equivalence of APs in topographically aligned 2D surfaces described here for neural space.

The least-time alignment of z spikes and photons make visual space topographically rigid at any instant, as tremor-synchronized spikes move in parallel (*Fig. 4.2*). The rhythmic wing beats of flocking birds, or sunlight flashing off the surface of schooling fish,[310] stimulate the synchrony of sustained retinotopic z spikes that gel the flock or the school into an elastic, holistic 3D organism.

Since here, spikes move instants of fixed emission times, comparison with successive instants of time is possible by concatenation of new spikes moving to the end of the neuron, where they evanesce, in a succeeding sequence. Sustained spikes thus tie together fixed instants of time synchronized at a sensory surface, with the passage of sequential time, so that sensed time is continuous due to the sequence of fixed emission times. A stable spike speed keeps sequential order, despite identical spike synchronization and serial synaptic summations. It is thought that the phase-locked firing of specifically timed input spikes retains the ordered timing of sequential peripheral stimuli within the slower theta rhythm.[311] What could be a disorderly state, due to varying stimulus intensities and spike rates, along with varied synaptic summation times, can cause spikes in parallel pathways to race competitively for ascendancy in perception. As already described, this occurs in metacontrast, where delayed perception attempts to order sequential retinal inputs of different areal intensities and axonal spike velocities in a convergently aligned z section. Dancers are able to synchronize movements, singers voices and birds

---

[310] Kowalko, J., Rohner, N., Rampani, S., Peterson, B., Linden, T., Yoshizawa, M., Kay, E., Weber, J., Hoekstra, H., Jeffery, W., Borowsky, R., Tabin, C. (2013) Curr. Biol. <u>23</u>:1874; vision is necessary to school.

[311] Panzeri et al., op. cit.

flocking behavior, via synapses in orthogonal x-y surfaces that synchronize latent percepts with the ongoing sequence of sustained RGC parallel spike inputs, as plotted in 2D time of *Fig. 4.2*. The phase-locked coordination of moving z time and repeated 2D surfaces extends across the body and its appendages, to varying distances and times, due to the initial impedance match of egocentric visual space gated at the retinal surface.

The impedance match of time and distance in 3D is exquisitely seen in dragonfly pursuit and capture of flies.[312] A sudden change in prey flight path is followed by ~4 msec delay for the dragonfly head to rotate and refoveate, followed by ~47 msec lag to redirect the flight path via the wings. At a distance, the targeted fly is a small spec on the dragonfly fovea and does not require reactive changes in flight path. As the fly looms on the fovea, rapid head reactions may become necessary, but are integrated within the stability of more delayed wing control, analogous to receptor precision synchronized with delayed cortical perception shown in *Fig. 4.2*. Z spikes sustained during pursuit realign dragonfly foveal receptors, or ommatidia, with the target within a few msec, via the x-y spatial precision of the downstream lobula. The short latency of spikes at the lobula is similar to that already described in the retinotopic SC, in which fixation cells redirect foveal targeting within milliseconds, without conscious cortical intervention and long circuit loops and delays, by comparison of small differences in x-y location of prey-stimulated z spikes. The short lag in head reaction as the prey image drifts on the dragonfly fovea awaits publication of neural routes. Anatomical

---

[312] Mischiati, M., Lin, H.-T., Herold, P., Imler, E., Olberg, R., Leonardo, A. (2015) Nature 517:333.

division of labor at serial 2D surfaces may have evolved circuitry for rapid accurate responses, or that rapidly learn and memorize predictive prey flight patterns, similar to the rapid reflexive behavior of flocking birds just described.

To take a different slant on the problem of temporal simultaneity in neurons, one must look to a diagram of the retina (*Fig. 4.3*). At a single instant, light from a distance of light-years arrives on the retinal surface at the same time as light emitted by an object 6 inches from the retina. This equivalence of all z distances at a single time at an orthogonal 2D surface is seen in 3D space only at the central optical z axis with its extended depth of field at all focal distances (*Figs. 3* and *4*). Linear perspective, accommodative focus, vergence and other factors (footnote 18) create perceived distance at one monocular surface. It seems paradoxical that light rays from

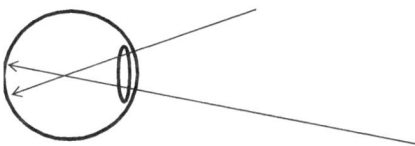

Fig. 4.3: Rays of light from expansive space geometrically converge the image on the 2D retina during fixation. However, a receptor cannot discriminate z distance or emitted time of aligned rays of identical photons when they impinge on the same 2D location on a retina. But the same ray arrival times at arrayed receptors are synchronized by FEMs, so the discrimination of various z distances at any synchronous x-y time occurs at convergent binocular V1/V2 cells. The perception of external proximal-distal 3D connectivity depends on this x-y FEM synchrony at any sequentially specific time. Any point in a monocular image has only one unobstructed origin, so differences in least-time spike arrival times from dual monocular spatial disparities at binocularly convergent V1/V2 cells, from the same external edge(s), synchronize a sense of stereoscopic x-y-z depth sustained by binocularly reemitted z spike times. Larger binocular RFs have aligned convergent synapses that reemit at the same rate as precisely synchronized inputs.

different distances and directions, with no preset temporal synchrony, form organized imagery on the retinal surface; however, tremor synchronizes precisely timed x-y snapshots during fixation. The shortest distance and least time for an impacting photon has one trajectory; perifoveal receptors filter out photons from the same spatial point with longer trajectories from different directions, helped by the Styles-Crawford effect cited in Chapter One.

That photons with different emission times corresponding to various distances in space, can impinge at the same time, at all locations on the orthogonal retinal surface, justifies the imposition of a synchronous instant of "clock time" on multiple z-aligned spikes at serial topographical x-y locations, as schematized in *Fig. 4.2*. The spike reemission at a binocular cell in response to synchronously timed monocular inputs (Read & Cumming, op. cit. Chapter One) makes static at each fixational tremor, both the retinal locations of the photons from the convergent distant point in the image and the temporally fused binocular percept that accrues over a fixation period of 150 msec. In other words, to perceptually connect distant and near space, the observer's brain sees spike latencies from distant locations in the same fixational time as spike latencies from near space, rather than in a later fixation. This necessity at the egocentric observer, to perceive both near and far space in each acausal instant of FEM induced x-y synchrony, has important implications for perceptions of the path taken by least-time light in space and also the expanding universe.

To create perceptions, neurons converge into larger RFs, demonstrating that simultaneous x-y time, of synchronized spikes impinging upon a spatially convergent neuron, transforms to emitted z spike time.

The direction of time can be simultaneous or sequential, depending on whether the observation is from a 2D surface facing the parallel inputs or at right angles to the inputs. In a spatially convergent neuron, the circuit itself has this orthogonality; simultaneous spikes in the x-y dimension become sequential spikes, but the precision of spike emission times are not lost as a rate code over time.[313] Here, z spikes are mobile instants of fixed emission times, which least-time synchronize at RF-aligned convergent synapses; due to the equivalence of synchronized identical spikes at all z distances, the delayed percept at cortex is simultaneous in time with fixationally sustained retinal spikes (*Fig. 4.2*). The FEM synchronization of RGC spikes is not lost at convergent neurons that reemit high frequencies rapidly in a time window of one or a few msec.[314]

At any rate, what is 'speed'? It is variable and transient, when locally measured at a specific time. But, greater distance from the observer's receptors is accompanied by greater latency, so distal speed seems slower. The observer's egocentric perspective of a distal focal point is dominated by expansive distal space, so that a distal point's distance/time ratio, in Gibsonian optical flow, scales the convergent local percept as distal smallness and slowness. The seeming stability of a large moving visual field relative to that of a local foveated point, is shown in Bridgeman et al. (1980, op. cit. Chapter Three). That distal speed is slower relative to local speed,

---

[313] Gutig, R., Gollisch, T., Sompolinski, H., Meister, M. (2013) PLoS One 8:e53063; Montemurro et al., op. cit.; higher sustained firing rates (above 100 Hz) converge at synapses to reemit precise spikes that preferentially phase-lock in a specific phase of longer duration cycles that compose a theta rhythm below 12 Hz.

[314] Pouille & Scanziani, Milstein et al., op. cit.; Mastronarde, Usrey & Reid, Schnitzer & Meister, Reinagle & Reid, all op. cit. Chap. Three.

requires that near and far parallaxes converge on a retinal surface, in which light from all distances impinges on a 2D sensor array at each sequential instant of time (*Fig. 4.3*). Light speed is a constant, in c = frequency * wavelength, due to the inversely related standardized units on the right side of this equation.[315] The egocentric observer perceives the variable local and distal on an orthogonal surface at the same time, as the same distance/latency ratio c, a constant if the light ray's emitted time is known.

The constancy of c at the observer is locally consistent with a slower distal optical flow, in which photons with longer distances/latencies converge to and synchronize at sequential times at the retinal surface. Increased intervals between spikes that correlate with increase in neural distance to larger RFs, show this expanded size of a time unit with increased distance in a constant ratio (*Fig. 5*), which stabilizes the perception of distal space via spike synchronies that enlarge RF area over z distance. If speed c is constant, distance (i.e. longer wavelength) has a proportional extension of its variable time unit (the associated slower frequency). Spike speed (distance/time) synchronizes spike frequency and latency at serially expanded RF areas (*Fig. 4.2*).

A recent report models the dynamics of spike initiation in a PYC axon, with the impedance load imposed by its dendritic arbor. Impedance increases with the neuron's dendritic surface area, which increases both the abruptness of the spike slope, and rapidity of spike initiation at the attached axon; in turn this causes output spikes to impedance match,

---

[315] Hecht, E. & Zajac, A. <u>Optics</u>, any edition. This equation has the same dimensional units (m/sec) as local speed v = distance/one-standard-time-unit, but differs in that the inverse proportionality keeps c constant, rather than a variable v due to invariant local time.

or phase-lock, with even higher frequencies of inputs.[316] This novel result came from the integration of the axonal spike initiation site and its dendritic field, previously separated in models. If an impedance match is required to phase-lock spikes, shouldn't it also be in larger interactions of retinal space-time and of external space-time?

The emitted time of a spike, which here is fixed as it moves at a constant distance/latency ratio to distal locations, is analogous to the fixed time retained by photons moving at speed c. If the observer moves at speed c, sequential time stops. A static emission time is necessary as a photon or spike moves over distance, so that the emission time does not include transit time but is solely the fixed time emitted at the initial location. Any instant of synchrony of proximal sustained spikes and distal perceptual spikes, fixes an emitted time that is intrinsic (without coding), as long as the spike moves. If tremor moves an orthogonal x-y surface, synchronizing edge-spikes, they spatially and temporally converge synchronously at univariantly active synapses, to z reemit rapidly. Sustained emitted times are distinguishable in relation to aging z spikes, despite convergence, because a spike's distance and latency are proportional at serial synapses that synchronize with spike reemission, as shown in *Fig. 4.2*.[317] While

---

[316] Eyal, G., Mansvelder, H., DeKock, C., Seger, I. (2014) J. Neurosci. 34:8063; the specific neurons modeled were PYCs in hippocampus and layers 2/3 of cerebral cortex. Phase-locking was observed in the simulation up to 200 Hz in rat and 600 Hz in humans. Milstein et al., op. cit. also show passing of high frequencies due to input synchrony.

[317] While RGC emitted times are due to object edges, rapid reemission of temporally synchronous spikes at spatially convergent synapses z-synchronizes proximal-distal time, in which cortically enduring z spikes from proximal information is subliminal unless synchronized in aligned RFs, as shown in *Figs. 3.3 and 4.2*. A moving spike's emitted time acquires a latent context due to neuronal distance.

spike speed is nominally distinguished from the static, proportional distance/time ratio repeated at each serial 2D surface, the fact that multiple spikes quickly synchronize over long axonal distances, phase-locking faster than the comparatively slow speed of a single spike traveling that distance,[318] means that multiple z spikes at stable speeds, adjust emitted intervals to phase-lock repeated x-y surfaces as a resonant 3D x-y-z entity.

To return to the constant speed c, if a Doppler redshift or reduction in frequency is measured, is this due to a measured speed or the increased volume of distal space?[319] Similar to a resonant cavity's size, the longer period of the wavelength measured instrumentally correlates with the egocentric sense that distal optical flow is a slower speed, or distance/time. The equation c = frequency * wavelength matches a distal redshift in wavelength with local light speed, or c, at a sensory surface. At the egocentric observer, the increase in 3D space also creates a decline in supernovae brightness used as a standard reference to measure distance. Confounded in the same z section of the egocentric observer, are the volume of distal resonant space measured by wavelength increase, and an acceleration of distal speed with increased radial distance, when measured in standard reference units of distance and time. Speed is locally measured and sensed, but spatially resonant frequencies and wavelengths are holistic; both are quantified in distance/time units. Spike rate also confounds dual

---

[318] Traub, R., Whittington, M., Stanford, I., Jefferys, J. (1996) Nature 383:621.

[319] Perlmutter, S. (2000), in Lepton and Photon Inter. at High Energies 1: 715; has a more detailed explanation of the cosmological redshift and the Hubble's Law diagram that base this paragraph's arguments.

measures as one rate; it does not distinguish stimulus looming speed from its larger size, or between saccade speed and saccade distance (discussed in the next chapter). If one travels to any location, c is invariant at any instrument that measures a photon's emitted and latent times at that location. But the percept at any stable local space and time, is that space has aged (or slowed), or time has an increased unit duration, due to wavelengths redshifting as space expands from the universe's birth. The temporal and spatial dimensions of the expanded universe are so large that the correlation between a receding supernova's measured brightness and redshift, expressed as Hubble's Law, cannot be perturbed to establish causation, but is solely a correlation, because the observer is a minute point in cosmological time. At any egocentric point limited in space and time, neurally distal space and near space are x-y correlated by FEM instants (*Fig. 4.3*), as is the division of labor in serial neural arrays in a perceptual moment[320] and synchronous z section (*Fig. 4.2*). Speed c matches at any synchronizing 2D surface, a constant distance/time ratio: of increased wavelengths over longer distances, with higher frequencies at short local distances. High frequencies impedance match with high RGC spike rates.

To belabor the point, Gibsonian optical flow diminishes drastically with distance to create distal spatial stability around the egocentric observer. This correlated scaling of slow distal optical flow with the cosmological redshift that stretches wavelength proportional to the expanded dimensions of distal space, both require an egocentric observer at a single fixational percept in time. In a single z section, an egocentric retina requires the proportional increase in

---

[320] Psychophysically dissected in Parise et al., op.cit.

3D distal space to be proportionally slower in frequency and older in time. This stable distant low-resolution space with a long time constant, and a stable distance/time c, scales to varying local speeds measured with standard units. If the observer or instrument was not a 2D surface at a convergent point in space and time, no expansion of the universe or of slow distal optical flow would be observable, as shown by the locally repetitive properties of 2D surfaces in *Fig. 2* of Chapter One. In addition, any instant of fixational time at the egocentric observer requires identical z spikes at repeated 2D surfaces (*Fig. 4.2*), for convergent perception to synchronize with varying receptor information.

The speed of light is constant, even if speeds at distal spatial locations are not directly measurable, due to locally invariant measurement of proportional distance/latency between the observer and any point in space. The astronomical inference is that due to homogeneous spatial properties, c is constant when measured anywhere. Constant speed c relative to the observer's motion has no directional bias in light reflected back to the local measuring apparatus. This homogenous lack of bias is the same as that shown by Hubble's uniform expansion of the universe. Together, these ideas inductively suggest that an egocentric 2D retina senses (or measures with a proxy instrument) a c speed that synchronizes with biological 1D z spikes at serially proportional distance/latency neural layers (as in Fig. 4.2).

A 3D spatial percept requires light to reduce frequency (increase wavelength) due to increased distance, to compatibly synchronize the latent distal with the immediate local 2D sensory surface (*Fig. 4.3*) at any instant of sequential time. The simultaneous percept of local and distal space in an egocentric z section, is matched with gamma frequencies, as shown in the schema of *Fig. 4.2*, of orthogonal, x-y synchronized RGC spike times, which converge fixationally sustained z spikes into reemitted latent z perception. The identical, data-neutral z spikes enable retinal image resolution to synchronize via least-time routing, from each 2D point in the visual image, via jittering cones, to RF-aligned foveal V1/V2 cells (*Fig. 3.3*).

Like the reduced speed and shorter wavelength of light upon entry into a medium that is measured as refractive index (RI), an impedance match of photons at c speed, transitions to RGC spikes with a low speed of several meters/sec. Single photons impedance match to the emission of single spikes.[321] RIs at the retina match light rays with specific receptor geometries.[322] One must posit that the measured spike speed of a few meters/sec is due to the standard units used to measure both spike and photon speeds. In reality, photon or spike speed, like wavelength or frequency, is intrinsic to the specific material, as is the RI. The variable time unit, or frequency, is due to differences in shape, elasticity, density, area, volume and other material properties. Quartz crystals, waveguides, resonant cavities, antennas and the expanded universe all have structures that specify resonant and harmonic frequencies.[323] A composite frequency or wavelength can have heterogeneous influences, or be due to homogenous, repeated elements.

---

[321] Barlow, H., Levick, W., Yoon, M. (1971) Vision Res. Suppl. 3:87.

[322] As Hecht & Zajac op. cit., show, rays of light bend more at shorter wavelengths; though light of normal incidence preferentially stimulates foveal cones, they accept light from larger incident angles than peripheral cones and rods, due to the Styles-Crawford effect.

[323] See Wikipedia entries for 'crystal oscillator' and 'wavelength'.

Analogous to a crystal's frequency, averaged cortical synchrony of spatially distributed oscillations is recorded from the synchronized reemission of inputs, in which spikes emit in phase from a group of neurons at the same time and location.[324] The transient shifting of RGC RF edges across image edges, stimulates rapidly reemitted LGN and V1 least-time z spikes. The percept is x-y stable, not due to 2D RF stability, but to simplify, because reemitted z spikes are convergent 1D locations/times that temporally synchronize with retinal x-y information. Only synchronized inputs stimulate convergent z spikes, so any univariant cell that reemits in the expanded cell populations that occupy serially larger RFs, can phase-lock proximal input spike rates with a phase of distal slower cortical theta rhythms.[325]

Thus stimulated synchrony of RGC, V1/V2 and V4 spikes, at high proximal-distal gamma frequencies, synchronizes perceptual 3D resolution with retinally fixated image edges.[326] This perceptual precision occurs with spatial convergence in aligned but larger RFs at LGN, V1/V2 and V4 levels, so that the collective edges of an object temporally synchronize cells in serial RFs (see *Fig. 4.6*). As discussed, unless

---

[324] Salinas & Sejnowski, op.cit.

[325] Univariance is from Li et al. op. cit. Chap. One. Alignment of receptor RF with cortical RF is necessary for a shorter latency response in the convergent cortical neuron. Phase-amplitude-rate coupling of gamma frequencies with theta rhythms is in Canolty, R., Edwards, E., Dalal, S., Soltani, M., Nagarajan, S., Kirsch, H., Berger, M., Barbero, N., Knight, R. (2006) Science 313:1626; also Panzeri et al., op. cit.

[326] Frien, A., Eckhorn, R., Bauer, R., Woelbern, T., Kehr, H. (1994) Neuroreport 5:2273; though V1 and V2 are sequential stages in primates, gamma rhythms phase-lock these stages. This is required for temporal and spatial resolution to synchronize as a proximal-distal stereo perception. Umeda et al., Shiozaki et al., op. cit. Chap. Three, also measure similar V1-V4 spike rates and resolution limits.

synchronously reemitted into long-duration z spikes, proximal mistimed or misaligned spikes do not re-emit and are subliminal. The x-y synchrony of RGCs transforms to z frequency as convergent reemissions occur in serial monocular and binocular RFs.

Because the analytically separate concepts of motion, location, emitted and enduring time are integrated in each z spike, but not as a standardized temporal code, each RGC emitted time moves as a micro-memory that stays fixed due to the proportional distance/latency created by its movement over distance. If z spikes did not also have temporally synchronized rapid summation and reemission at convergent synapses (which is also due to equal input latencies), serial visual stages of spatial summation would lose RGC edge-timed precision. This is affirmed by perceptually measured categorization and identification scores of stimuli, correlating with the fastest one or two spikes at spatially convergent clusters of IT cells.[327] The initial FEM-synchronized RGC spike emission times are feature-selected serially by the most rapid convergent reemissions to specific groups of IT cells that selectively respond to, and thus categorize the stimulatory features.

The extremely rapid onset of gamma synchronization by initial z spikes indicates this synchrony is more important than the slower increase in rate coding, to categorize stimuli.[328] While research tries

---

[327] Hung et al. op. cit. Chap. Three.

[328] Maldonado et al., op. cit.; Ito, J., Maldonado, P., Singer, W., Grun, S. (2011) Cereb. Cort. 21:2482; phase-locking of initial spikes in V1 occurred 40-60 msec after fixation onset, 20 msec before the peak firing rate. This phase-lock time was not dependent on informational differences of detailed images vs. blank images, so does not encode image information. However, higher edge contrast and image detail increase spike rates and frequencies for greater timing precision.

to find the biophysical and causal basis for this 'anticipatory synchronization' in serial synapses,[329] it may be a process of 'z equivalence' hypothesized here. This equivalence requires an invariant neural distance/spike latency ratio at serial synapses, also known as spike speed, synchronized with spike rate. This creates a 3D integration of synchronous 1D z spikes with x-y aligned topography. A stable distance/time ratio synchronizes moving spike loci with stationary loci; if average spike rate is analyzed as specific distance/time intervals, RF-aligned z spikes at serial loci will have no phase lag. Identical 1D z spikes are present at sequential distances/times in aligned 2D arrays as shown in *Fig. 4.2*; so does proximal-distal synchrony at any sequential instant, replace multiplexing and subsequent decoding of peripheral information at a distal location?

A traditional spike latency code depends on temporal differences in the pattern of RGC inputs corresponding to the shape of a stimulus.[330] The summation time that initiates the first emitted spike is a characteristic that varies with the RGC type; it also varies with the proportion of stimulated Off and On bipolar cells that input to the RGC. Differences in the convergent summation time also result if the whole RF or part of the RF is stimulated by the object shape. This has been interpreted to mean that RGC latency differences in the orthogonal x-y plane encode stimulus off-on areas, thus the stimulus pattern. But here the timing of spike inputs at a convergent cortical synapse is not determined by stimulus-specific latencies, but on the FEMs that

---

[329] Traub et al., op. cit.; does this rapid synchronization require identifying information in each serial spike, or are spikes identical?

[330] Gollisch, T., Meister, M. (2008) Science: $\underline{319}$:1108; Gutig, R., Gollisch, T., Sompolinsky, H., Meister, M. (2013) PLoS One $\underline{8}$:e53063.

emit RGC spikes in a short time window, which then temporally and spatially synchronize at univariant synapses in serial stages. Peripheral small receptor RFs impedance match edge-stimulated emitted times with external stimulus information, as previously described. Where clusters of neurons respond to convergent features in distal IT cortex, 1D z synchronies have increased to dominate via increased latency and duration, subliminal latency differences reemitted by peripheral RGCs. As Hung et al. have shown, the fastest z spikes temporally and spatially synchronize in IT cortex, which correlates with high behavioral accuracy in categorizing and identifying stimulus object features; this is due to a short 12.5 msec time window of spike coincidence in clustered IT cells, not retinal latency differences, while fixationally sustained spikes still emit from RGCs.

As stated here, proximal-distal z synchrony of fixationally sustained RGC output, phase-locks FEM frequencies with z gamma frequencies throughout the serial retinotopically aligned RFs of the visual system. Distal perceptual rhythms may periodically skip emitted times sustained proximally by the same edge pattern, whose z locations, but not coded x-y information, anatomically and temporally converge to IT cells from any x-y location in the visual field. The least-time distal IT 1D z spikes, fix the object feature spike times emitted by RGCs, via a reemitted latent synchronous convergence that matches proximal FEM spike synchrony with distal z spikes (*Fig. 4.2*) in serial, x-y aligned cell RFs.

To review previous assertions, the simultaneous orthogonal x-y perception of distant and near space (indicated in *Fig. 4.3*) synchronizes with a constant serial ratio of distance/time on z axes. This relationship of longer wavelengths with slower frequencies, matches the redshift of expanded space to the observer's egocentric time and location. The notion of a 'big bang' results, in which the most distant supernovae emit light of the longest wavelength, and thus the largest recession distance/time, even though distal space has the same homogeneous properties as local space if the observer travels there. The egocentric observer requires local and distal space to have x-y RGC spike synchrony and synchronized z spike frequencies in each proximal-distal z section, otherwise the physical connectivity of near and far space is not perceived.[331]

The perspectival image that results because light rays from distal 3D space impinge onto 2D retinal surfaces, is bypassed when coherent 1D laser light stimulates receptors on the retinal surface, which creates interference fringes with a perceived resolution on the order of a wavelength of light. This resolution is much higher than that of ordinary light rays that converge via the eye's optics through the cornea, lens and the vitreous and aqueous humors onto the retina.[332] Similarly immune from degradative effects is laser speckle on the retina, which results from wave interference when the normally phase-coherent laser light reflects or refracts from a relatively rough external surface onto the retina. The direction in which the speckle moves as the perceiver moves, indicates how well the perceiving eye's optics are focused on a distant point, though

---

[331] Paradoxically, if wavelength expands proportionally with distance in space, to create a redshift interpreted as an increase in recession velocity (velocity is a vector quantity, integrating speed and direction) at the same c speed, does this dilated distal wavelength actually cause a reduced velocity of redshifted wavelengths (measured as phase velocity, defined in footnote 345) at the egocentric observer? This lower phase velocity is consistent with dilated (or slower) distal unit time.

[332] Williams, D. (1985) J. Opt. Soc. Am. A $\underline{2}$:1087.

the speckle itself is not focusable.[333] The distal wave superpositions or interference fringes that are perceived as retinal speckle, also do not have an image instability caused by FEMs, but must be a property limited by 2D surface impedance matching, because speckle moves with the perceiver in the x-y plane, but does not have perspectival effects caused by perceiver movements on the z axis, which is consistent with anatomical z distance equivalence normal to repeated 2D surfaces described here. Quantum mechanical 'entanglement' has a similar distance equivalence at synchronized times. Entanglement phenomena may be physically reified sensory orthogonal x-y planes, which are fundamental to perceptual synchronies in each z section.

Perceived time is necessarily correlated with spatial distance, as in the Pulfrich illusion, in which perception to one eye of an object swinging back and forth across the field of view, is artificially delayed by a filter or lens (or temporarily absent if a strobed stimulus is used to simulate the delay) so is stereoscopically seen to bow inward and outward in orthogonal trajectory due to the slower speed of filtered light to that eye's z axis.[334] This reciprocal space-time duality, of perceived distance versus perceived speed, is an indirect result of stimulated motion-sensitive RGCs that rapidly emit identical, successive z spikes with no coded x-y information, but respond to x-y aligned timing of inputs in least time. These 1D z spikes temporally summate, and temporally correlate, with the external location of

---

[333] The speckle phenomenon applied to human visual optics is described in Saleh, B. (1982) in <u>Applications of Optical Fourier Transforms,</u> Stark, H. ed., p. 431.

[334] See Read & Cumming op. cit. Chap. One, for a detailed discussion of neuronal timing in the Pulfrich illusion from monocular inputs.

the moving object, at convergent synapses that impedance match synchronously to the visual field location. With temporal delay in one eye, the proportionality of distance/time corresponds to a bowing-in of object location as it speeds toward that eye, when perceived as reemitted z output from temporal spike synchrony at binocular cells. The rapidly reemitted response of the convergent synapses on these cells synchronously matches, in the same z section, with the external object location. The monocularly slowed speed over the short thickness of the filter (or imposed stroboscopic delay) is enough to change the location and timing of spike binocular convergence so that it is perceived larger and closer.

But the delayed photons that exit the filter resume their normal speed to the retina. The fact that we see the slowed speed and larger image at the distant filter location, although the photons have resumed normal speed near the retina, indicates that photons synchronize and impedance match from all 3D distances (*Fig. 4.3*), at successive, simultaneous times on the 2D retinal surface, reemitting 1D z spikes in each z section (*Fig. 4.2*), so that each z synchronous percept succeeds the previous one.

Causally, we know that photons flow in sequence to the retina, but because they have no rest mass, they have instant speed, with no hysteresis between photons. This temporal and spatial rigidity is similar to a moving sequence of z spikes. The Pulfrich illusion, with a filtered or strobed delay at one retina, causes an altered parallax perception of movement due to z synchrony in binocular cells that are in x-y synchrony with the undelayed stimulus at the other retina. If the monocular delay is in a sequential later z section, rather than a delayed binocular percept in the same z section, this would create a veridical, non-illusional perception of stimulus location and speed, but perceived delayed in sequence.

How does least-time work, if so many latencies of converging photons (and spikes) are present? The constant speed of photons or spikes is a distance/time constraint that is a natural consequence of the sequential order of stimulation. This sequentiality is preserved in the refractive change from air to a glass medium that reduces light speed, or physiologically, in the impedance change to RGCs with slower spike speeds. The last, largest cortical RFs have a delay within a z section that perceptually selects, or convergently filters, only the input spikes that RF-align within the shortest least-time neural route. Following the course of the spike emitted at '1' during the synchronous perceptual moment in Fig. *4.2*, shows that its eventual perceptual latency only accepts a properly ordered sequence of an edge's emitted-time spikes, at convergent synapses in the cortical x-y aligned RF. In other words, synchronous summation at longer latency convergent, perceptual synapses aligns *retroactively* during each z section with newly sustained inputs, to filter, via recurrent inhibition, a least-time order from spike fixed emission times. The least-time increase in speed and distance of light trajectory induced by a mirage (discussed in footnote 292), as also the reduced speed of light from air to glass or to spikes in a neuronal medium, are due to synchronization of emitted spike times at RGCs. Emitted spike times impedance match serial latencies and distances at each orthogonal 2D array of RF neurons, to also synchronize each proximal-distal z section.

The convergence of cone outputs upon RGCs, LGN cells and then the larger RFs of V1 cells (*Fig. 3.3*) shifts the spike route during tremor, as the external reference light ray aligns the shortest, strongest, fastest spike path emitted by an external high contrast image edge. Synchronized spikes emphatically reemit from contrasty edges.[335] Identical spikes at serially aligned 2D locations are present at the same time, so that these z locations on each x-y aligned neural route have z equivalence during synchrony.[336] Compare to a camera with a fast shutter that takes a succession of still images with reconstructed information in each one. Here, each FEM-gated retinal shift triggers synchronous RGC spikes, which are in gamma synchrony with cells throughout the depth of columns in visual cortex.[337] X-y synchronized RGC spikes race to any equidistant, RF aligned, univariant synapse. It is this serially reemitted temporal synchronization, in the distance/time of the z dimension, which endures latently as a stable percept of z-synchronized, subliminal shifting of x-y RFs. The convergent 1D z spikes reemitted, create a longer duration of intrinsic z image stability despite minimized V1 RFs that jitter at high frequency. A reiteration of retinotopy in larger cortical RFs does not x-y stabilize retinal imagery, but is serially perceived as synchronous z spikes. Activated perceptual RFs reemit z spikes that filter through convergent synapses in modular arrays into longer distance/time synchrony. One may test that synaptically reemitted z spikes in activated RFs are perceptual, rather than the orthogonal RF x-y shifting by differentiating 1D z time from x-y properties.

---

[335] Laughlin, S. (1989) J. Exp. Biol. 146:39; argues that visual neurons code contrast alone, to the exclusion of other information; here edge contrast creates more precise emission times at RF edges.

[336] Mizuseki & Buzsaki, op. cit.; spike synchrony moves no information, here due to the repetition in space and time of identical spikes.

[337] Welle, C., Contreras, D. (2016) J. Neurophys. 115:1821; Llinas, R., Leznik, E., Urbano, F. (2002) PNAS (USA) 99:499.

To be more anatomically specific, the corticofugal outputs from V1 simple cells select, or synaptically filter, the sequential spikes from convergent LGN outputs, via RF matching of serial 2D surfaces (*Fig. 4.2*). The latent awareness of object features and stability results from 1D z spike synchronization from convergent labeled neurons rather than multi-dimensional multiplexed image information. LGN input to V1 cortex, at 15-30 Hz, reemits at a lower rate, in the 8-14 Hz alpha rhythm, from V1 cortex back to LGN, hypothetically due to differing resonant impedance matches along axonal and dendritic trees.[338] Because RGC output sustains, convergent latent cortical perception not only was caused by prior inputs, but also synchronizes with subsequent inputs during the fixation period. Convergent re-emitted z spikes endure over the neural distance from retina to IT cortex for the 120-150 msec perceptual moment (*Fig. 5* applied to *Fig. 4.2*). During fixation, edge-precise RGC spike micro-memories fire in a gamma rhythm synchronous with a specific phase of a slower frequency such as the cortical alpha rhythm, which signals perceptual variations in detectability of stimuli. The alpha rhythm overlaps with the frequency ranges of cortical and hippocampal theta rhythms.[339]

To recap, only emitted spikes that impinge on convergent synapses within aligned RFs synchronously, reemit as z spikes into latent cortical perception, which is an impedance match with external image

---

[338] Bastos et al., op. cit. Chap. Three.

[339] Mathewson, K., Gratton, G., Fabiani, M., Beck, D., Ro, T. (2009) J. Neurosci. 29:2725; Garrido, M., Barnes, G., Kernavan, D., Maguire, E., Dolan, R. (2015) Neuroimage 128: 361; Canolty et al. and Montemurro et al., op. cit.; alpha and theta rhythms overlap the same frequency range (depending on the reference), but are nominally different due to different sources of stimulation.

edges. Because this process matches spike rate with the spike latency to specific synapses in serial arrays, the repeated traversal of 1D z spikes over longer distances at slower reemitted rates and frequencies results in a resonantly stable, phase-locked temporal and spatial percept that preserves peripheral precision without averaging or multiplexing information, as current methods may suggest.

The orthogonal combination of spatial convergence on serial RFs and a synchronous z section (so that multiple fixed times of identical spikes transiently pass proximal-distal RFs in serial stages), requires a least-time photon and spike route to synchronize sequential spike micro-memories at serial RFs from the same image edge. In *Fig. 4.4* following, the drift of an object edge across the retinal surface converges the same spike emitted times into alignment from feature selective RGCs to V1 RFs,[340] and into proximal-distal z synchrony at terminal IT cells.

How else does phase-locked perception affect objective physics? A source of light diverges to multiple organismal synchronized z sections, which in physics, are interpreted as parallel universes.[341] The observer's orientation with respect to a trajectory of spikes determines whether synchronous waves or a temporal sequence of spikes is seen; in physics, wave-particle duality is similar in concept. A plane with double slits placed in a coherent stream of photons, with a following parallel plane to show wave

---

[340] Kagan et al., op. cit. Chap. Three; V1 cells responsive to FEMs may be of two types; those that transiently respond to microsaccades or those with sustained responses at slower drift speeds. The increase in V1 spike rate to either type occurs after a transient dip in rate, or saccadic suppression, in the first 50-100 msec after the FEM initiates.

[341] See <u>Our Mathematical Universe</u>, by Tegmark, M. (2014), which duscusses the hypothesis of multiple universes in parallel.

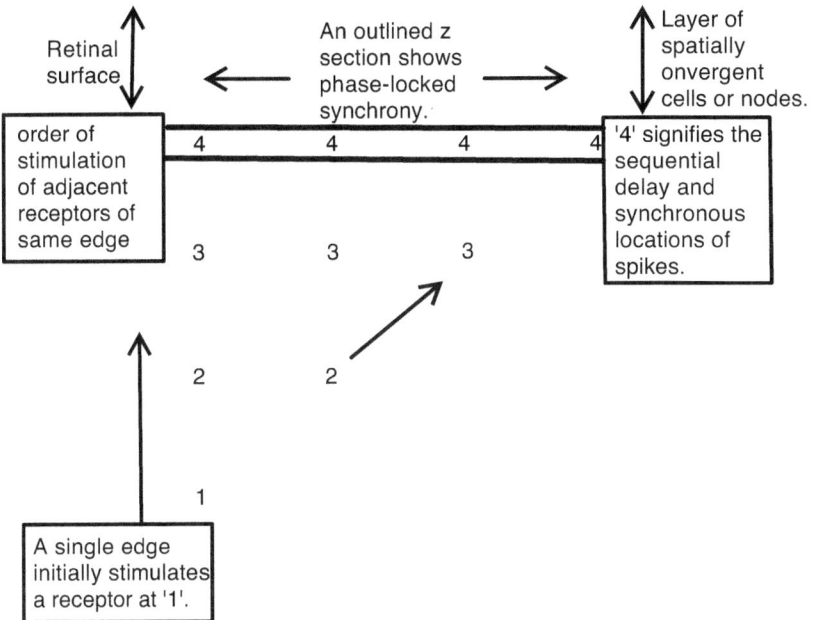

Fig. 4.4: This variant of Fig. 4.2 illustrates how spatial convergence from adjacent receptors, of sustained spikes from the same stimulus edge that crosses adjacent RGC RF edges, develops proximal-distal z-axis synchrony. Number sequence denotes latency order. Z spikes of the same latency align for synchrony in the same z section that becomes x-y sequential across adjacent z sections. So what is construed by the external observer as an edge drifting randomly across retinal receptors, is actually aligning the same edge-emitted latency at serial synapses. A slow drift speed across the retinal surface synchronizes with convergent summation latencies at serially reemitting synapses in this model. Half of a 2D layer of convergent inputs is shown. This model scales to 3D, from receptors to RGCs to following 2D layers of synapses, which reemit identical z spikes that converge and temporally synchronize via increasing numbers of serial, feature-selective labeled synapses in larger RFs, to convergent IT cells in clusters.

interference, allows visualization of the cumulative formation of waves by photons in the plane orthogonal to their trajectory.[342] The interference of

---

[342] This phenomenon is like ergodic theory, in which the measurements at one spatial location averaged over time, are equivalent to those over many spatial locations averaged at a single point in time.

waves that are spatially distributed on an orthogonal plane in this double-slit experiment, "undo" their spatially correlated interference backward in time if one can determine which slit individual photons traveled through.[343] This time reversal by individual particles whose impacts form interference fringes over time, may be sourced in synchronized z spikes, which have no tag or time code, except the continuously emitted fixed times constituting each 1D synchronous z section. The orthogonal axes of 2D time in *Figs. 4.2-4.4* visualize both synchronous and sequential time (analogous to wave-particle duality and the simultaneous 0 and 1 states of quantum entanglement, mentioned earlier). Recent theory requires multiple time dimensions for symmetry considerations in quantum mechanics.[344]

The necessary binding of a time dimension to every spatial dimension in the expostulation here, impedance matches and integrates perceptual synchrony with external physics, based on neuronal anatomy and spike emission times and latencies. For the theory here, one must have a robust understanding of neuronal properties before adding layers of intuitive physical theory, which in a recursively complex way, attempt to explain external physical reality that intrinsic neuronal mechanisms have understood for eons. These neuronal mechanisms summate into long-latency perceptual moments, requiring that visual reality is constrained to be a complete percept at the minimal latency required to synchronize each z section. Therefore each z section requires physical constants that impedance match within the limits

---

[343] For more details of the delayed choice quantum eraser experiment, see Scully, M., Kim, Y-H., Kulik, S., Shih, Y.(2000) Phys. Rev. Lett. 84:1.

[344] Bars, I. & Kuo, Y. (2007) Phys. Rev. Lett. 94:041801.

imposed by the synchrony of the physical and neurophysiological at sensory 2D interfaces.

In the physical realm, light transmitted through an optically dense material, results in a slower light speed and shorter wavelengths, which, when light leaves the material at normal incidence angle to enter the eye, telescopes, or shortens, distance in the image so that the distal is perceived to be closer and larger in the same fixational percept.[345] Light delayed in the material still x-y synchronizes at the retinal surface with parallel light rays that bypass the material in the same synchronous percept, causing the successive instants of x-y synchrony at the retinal surface to be perceived with the delayed instants. If hypothetically delayed into a later z section, rather than perceived in the same z section, the delayed part of the image may not impedance match at the same synchronous time, but later in perceived time.

Cortically enduring 1D z spikes 'fix' by rapid reemission, neurally linked, proximal spike emitted times, as proximal-distal z-equivalent synchronized percepts of high gamma rhythm resolution in each successive z section. Convergent lower spike rates at distal cortical synapses may lack the information resolution of RGC spike rates, but here, the spike emitted times with receptor resolution are still sensed, via transient, univariantly shifting synchronizations of reemitted, identical 1D z spikes that

---

[345] This light delay is consistent with the physiological neural delay of the Pulfrich Illusion. See also Wikipedia entry for 'Refractive Index'. High RI light has a shorter wavelength and slower velocity in a material (according to the equation phase velocity = c/RI) so has the same synchronous (impedance matched) frequency within the material as external to it. The result is that both refracted (or phase delayed) and straight image light transmitted through a material are perceptually synchronous during fixation.

move location/time as a continual process, but not to a central decoding location. The moving z spikes *are* locations, so acquiring latency via successive spatially and temporally synchronous reemissions, which 1D z synchronize perceptual neurons in IT cortex with retinal multidimensional information.

The synchronization of external stimulation and the neural perceptual systems, requires serial matching, so that the measured impedance between each stage is minimized;[346] impedance matching is consistent with the Anthropic Principle,[347] in which physical constants necessary for life to exist are at precisely the values sensed by synchronized perceptual moments. The 2D time axes of *Figs. 4.2* and *4.4* show that external proximal-distal physical reality has to synchronize, or impedance match, with each FEM-synchronous instant of emitted z time.

The delay of visual perception as it reacts to stimulated spikes from labeled receptors, is conventionally explained as closed loop negative feedback with temporally coded information. Instead here, iterated topographical maps converge lagging spikes from proximal off-target x-y locations to an intended distally-mapped target; the synergism facilitates reemission of convergent least-time z spikes (*Figs. 4.2* and *4.4*). A resonant neural 3D requires anatomical typing of proximal receptors and neurons to prevent conmingling of external feature detail by identical

---

[346] See Wikipedia entry for 'Resonance'. Here, resonance is operationally defined as synchrony. Resonance is a complex property of membranes, ionic currents, impedance amplitude and phase of oscillation; more detail is in Hutcheon, B. & Yarom, Y. (2000) Trends Neurosci. $\underline{23}$:216. Variable impedance along a dendritic tree selects, or tunes, for resonant frequency, in Das, A., Rathour, R., Narayanan, R. (2017) Front. Cell. Neurosci. $\underline{11}$:72.

[347] Livio, M. & Rees, M. (2005) Science $\underline{309}$:1022.

spikes, filtered through increasing numbers of convergent, feature-selective synapses, which reemit 1D z spikes in a constant ratio of increasing locations/times. This constant ratio synchronizes spike speed and emitted rate with the latency and distance between linked synapses. What seems to be a dissonant concert of varied rhythms, is here a synchronization of specific distal and proximal neural locations, via intrinsic emitted and emergent latent times of continuously sustained spikes. Reduced spike rates due to serial synaptic reemissions are a result not of sparse coding of repetitive information, but of sustained, identical RGC spikes that synchronize during the fixation period even with substantially reduced spike rates; also a reduced spike frequency synchronizes z locations due to increased neuronal distances to distal synapses.

While Figs. *4.2* and *4.4* are based on the retinal motion of a single edge across receptors, can multiple edges comprising a whole object, as a 3D stereogram, be pictured with neural synchrony (*Fig. 4.5*)? FEM-generated emission times of spikes by all the edges that make up a shape, selected by convergent spatial and temporal synchronization at synapses, reemit the gamma rhythm synchronized with fixational retinal tremor. Because binocular V1/V2 cells respond to the same stimulus edge from dual monocular x-y locations, reemission may occur at any univariant binocular cell from any monocular RGC emissions synchronized by equal spike latency. But the averaged recordings from a specific binocular cell are to multiple disparities of the same stimulus edge that shift maximal response and alter spike rate,[348] contributing to the idea that binocular cell

---

[348] Cumming, B. & Parker, A. (2000) J. Neurosci. 29:4758; Tanabe et al. (2011) op. cit. Chap. Three.

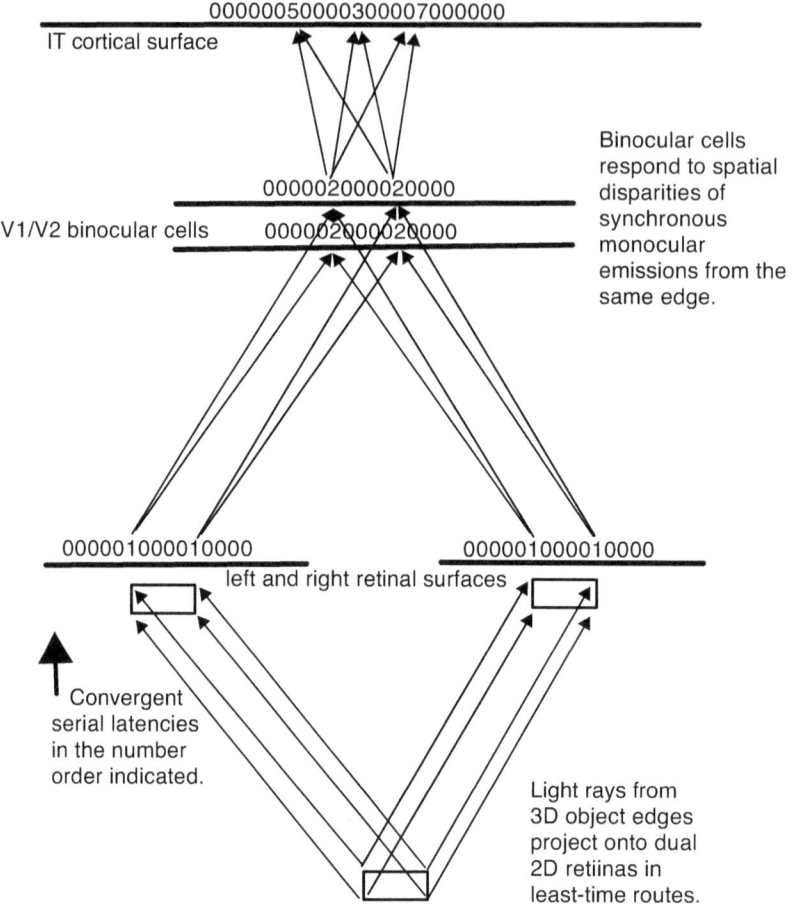

Fig. 4.5: RGC spikes orthogonally synchronized by FEMs, converge and diverge to LGN, SC, V1, V2, ..., and IT synapses in serial 2D arrays. Shape edge patterns synchronously emit RGC spikes that least-time converge to univariant binocular V1/V2 synapses, to reemit to V3, V4 arrays that perceive shapes, while movement sequentially stimulates spikes that filter through the same convergent circuits in V1/V2 to motion-perceiving V5 cortex. That stimulus edges emit spikes that synchronize at spatially convergent synapses in cortical perceptual areas, indicates that z spike times synchronize at proximal-distal 2D arrays, rather than multiplex spatial retinal precision as a transmitted code distally. The proximal-distal 3D perceptions of continuous spatial stability and continuous motion synchronize the same z spike locations, which distally summate most rapidly in multiple IT cells as 1D z times that are both an internal perception and external observation.

populations respond with many 'false matches'. The binocular cell that responds with different maximal rates to different spatial disparities, is also signaling variable vergence angles of the eyes on varying focal distances.[349] These population responses are typically recorded as averages over time, but here, sequential instants of spatial and temporal synchronization proximally-distally, are actually most important for rapidly reemitted binocular perception. The spikes reemitted by multiple convergent synapses within retinotopically aligned but larger RFs of binocular cells, here do not multiplex information; but as identical mobile z locations, they converge at clusters of IT cells in least-time with increased spike rates as the correctly synchronized stereogram is perceived.[350] The increased distal spike rate increases precision of 3D stereo perception at specific IT cells. The image is not distally reconstructed in 3D, but x-y synchronized spike latencies rapidly reemit proximal-distal convergent z spikes; this distributed x-y-z synchrony *is* stereo perception in any sequential z section visualized at a static time.

A recent model of 3D vision, using neuromorphic chips, converges on some aspects of the theory described here.[351] In this other version, time and location are tagged onto each stimulated edge event, rather than as an average or programmed sequence, so are asynchronously timed information packets, stimulated by specific external events, with

---

[349] Trotter et al. (1996) op. cit. Chap. Three; the mean latency from three focal distances (or three binocular vergence angles) had a peak value of 60 msec in the population of V1 cells recorded.

[350] Janssen, P., Vogels, R., Liu, Y., Orban, G. (2003) Neuron 37:693.

[351] Osswald, M., Ieng, S-H., Benosman, R., Indiveri, G., (2017) Sci. Rprts. 7:40703; simplifying data and modeling to recreate binocular vision in computational systems also creates more insight.

terminal addresses. These addressed packets traverse coincidence detectors, then disparity detectors, to be decoded as image objects on a 3D depth map serially in time. Their model works with precise temporal contrast, but does not use spatial contrast, composed of orientation, spatial frequency or spatial disparity information, or sustained spike events, so is similar to the M system of neurons. In their model, near synchronous inputs reemit from disparity detectors for 3D vision; inhibitory V1 interactions also sharpen the reconstructed stereo image.[352]

The theory here differs, because rather than using asynchronous edge-events tagged with location and time codes, edge-emitted time is intrinsic to the moving spike (*Fig. 4.1*); the rapid reemission at binocular synapses 'remember' the monocular sensor fixed emitted times by the synchronized frequencies and latent wavelengths of spikes repetitively reemitted at serial spatially and temporally convergent synapses. In the theory here, no x-y tags or data are calibrated, reconstructed or coded by identical 1D z spikes; the proximal-distal synchronization in each sequential z section correlates the latent 1D z time of perception with the multidimensional quality of each proximal event time (*Fig. 4.2*). Tags or codes are necessary for digitally clocked processing but not for the proximal-distal z synchrony here.

Binocular cell spike rates are due to two independent parameters, spatial x-y disparity and temporal z spike summation.[353] Serial topographically mapped

---

[352] Tanabe, Haefner et al., op. cit. Chap. Three.

[353] Read & Cumming, op. cit. Chap. One, their Fig. 3; in other words, the reemitted binocular response to equally timed monocular inputs does not jointly modify the retinotopic x-y spatial disparity responsiveness.

arrays and moving z spike locations at specific z times, require multiple electrode arrays in the visual pathway to adequately analyze the synchrony of emitted and reemitted spikes. The peak rate of the fastest-response binocular V1/V2 cell has more precision than adjacent cells responsive to spatial and temporal non-zero disparities from the same monocular receptors, a population of 'false matches'. But the adjacent V1/V2 cells must have comparable precise peak spike rates to the least-time mapped receptors adjacent to the reference receptor.

These least-time reemitted z spikes become perceptual due to endurance over time, impedance matching the extended z dimension with FEM-generated x-y synchrony. The latent binocular z response has little conventional information, but synchronizes with RGC spikes. This division of labor, of transiently aligned proximal monocular spikes that reemit binocular precision as already described, is perceived during sustained fixation as synchronized 3D depth. Assuming that massive computation of multiplexed data is occurring in cortex and to get a reliable signal, experimenters average this seemingly noisy precision to create heterogeneous data of extreme complexity and stochastic ambiguity.

In lieu of high quality data from multiple electrode arrays, or the heuristic shorthand that facilitates computer models, here sensory topographically-mapped serial surfaces avoid multidimensional coding by aligning 2D RFs, so that 1D z spikes synchronize the same repeated x-y locations. The temporal synchrony of proximal sustained and distal 1D z spikes (*Fig. 4.4*) avoids temporal encoding of image information to a perceptual location. Perceptual confounds are avoided because detailed spatial image information remains at receptors in a division of neural labor; variable edge information remains peripheral during saccades, while temporal convergence of z spikes in a distal IT cell cluster latently synchronizes with RGC stimulated spikes, so does not decode shifty x-y data for a distal stable image.

The same x-y precise z section has a specific receptor spatial resolution that emits spikes at rates that have temporal resolution; distal cortical stages that converge and reemit at lower spike rates perceive edge direction.[354] Within a range of drift speeds and changes in direction across the retina during fixation, an edge stimulates sustained spikes that reemit at serially convergent synapses. This convergence of spikes of the same latency (*Fig. 4.4*) is required so that convergent and inhibitory circuits create temporal lags between reemitted z spikes that synchronously oscillate in a narrow frequency range.[355] As discussed earlier, the degree of phase shift in an average frequency is relative to the cortical 3D location of a phase-locked frequency. During the fixation period, distal cortical RF-aligned spikes reemitted from the sequential drift of an edge across RGCs, synchronize with fixed emission times of spikes orthogonally synchronized at the retina by tremor. Sustained RGC emitted times correlate in a specific phase of distal reemitted spike frequencies.

---

[354] If one presumes a single RGC encodes a drifting edge, the intervals in its spike rate are too long to code directional edge motion across its convergent cone RFs; stated in Burak, Y., Rokni, U., Meister, M., Sompolinsky, H. (2010) PNAS (USA) <u>107</u>:19525. The central cortical decoding and computation of direction is replaced here with serial stages of x-y-z proximal-distal synchronization of repeated instants of z precision (*Fig. 4.4*) emitted in the high spike rate of RGCs.

[355] Brovelli, A., Ding, M., Ledberg, A., Chen, Y., Nakamura, R., Bressler, S. (2004) PNAS <u>101</u>:9849; sequential temporal lags between spikes, measured as Granger causal peaks, correlate with peak synchronized frequencies best in the 20-23 Hz range between macaque sensory-motor cortical areas.

The collective edges making up an object emit spikes that are spatially and temporally synchronized with the gamma rhythm of cells in serial arrays of repeated circuit modules. Here, spikes have intrinsic qualities of sequential, emitted and latent time that synchronize if identical z spikes continuously move in a proximal-distal integrated context. The intrinsic times of 1D z spikes, with no data tags, acquire abstract contextual properties simply due to synaptic convergence and reemitted duration, without multiplexing information, but synchronously timed and phase-locked with proximal information (*Fig. 4.6*). Spikes filter through serially selective

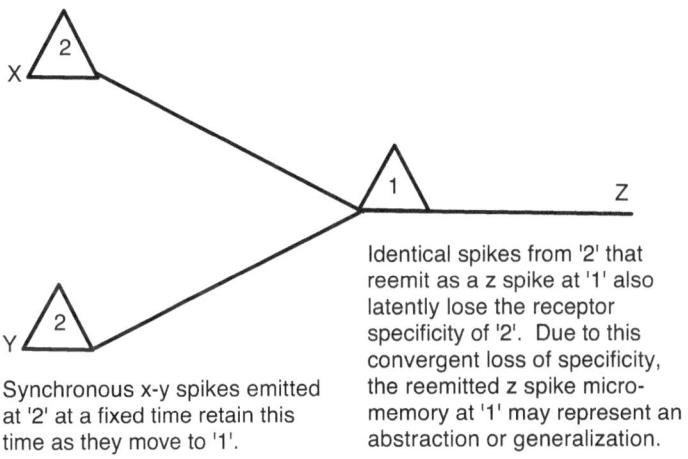

Synchronous x-y spikes emitted at '2' at a fixed time retain this time as they move to '1'.

Identical spikes from '2' that reemit as a z spike at '1' also latently lose the receptor specificity of '2'. Due to this convergent loss of specificity, the reemitted z spike micromemory at '1' may represent an abstraction or generalization.

Fig. 4.6: The analysis of generic time into emitted, reemitted, sequential and synchronous times emerge as a spike moves in varying contexts. The same spike that emits with high RGC temporal resolution may reemit as distal 1D z temporal stability. FEMS shift RFs, as at '2', which converge monocular spikes at gamma frequencies to reemit at '1' at the same frequencies, in a convergent binocular RF. Temporal synchronization of x-y emitted and reemitted 1D z spikes, causes stable proximal-distal (RGC to IT) stereo percepts at each sequential emitted time. Sustained spikes enable emitted and reemitted z spike times to be perceived synchronously at sequential times, without averaging over time. In this serial circuit, z outputs reemit from converged x-y inputs in repetitive, cascaded arrays of neurons that possess increasingly larger RFs.

modular synaptic circuits, activating cortical areas with selective perceptual qualities, steered via least-time paths to recognition-specific clusters of IT cells.

CONCLUSIONS

1) Synchronization of z spike inputs at serial stages of orthogonal neural arrays is due to similar spike travel times to convergent synapses, properties which cause the selective reemission of onward spikes. Rather than a latency code that reconstructs retinal information, tremor frequency fixes the peripheral micro-memories, or emitted times, of the image in the continued synchronized reemission of spikes that move z location rather than detailed x-y information itself. These emitted-time micro-memories are an indiscriminate population response that converges and endures distally, if selectively reemitted from any synapse that rapidly summates inputs. The distal timing of spikes at serially convergent synapses, during the coinciding durations of both fixation and the perceptual moment, synchronizes with proximal retinal sustained spike rates that have high temporal and spatial resolution.

2) A z section constitutes an edge-stimulated repetitive sequence of spikes that summate at succeeding synapses, which, due to spatial and temporal summation, reemit fewer spikes at each stage. In other words, any emitted spike rate from an array correlates neural distance, spike latency and speed to serially synchronize at any reemitting synapse. However an exception exists in the stages of the visual system, which, stimulated by proximal-

distal gamma z spike frequencies, spatially integrate spike inputs from monocular retinotopic arrays for the exacting precision of 3D stereopsis. Serial spatial and temporal convergence and filtering of spikes at synapses, overlap in time to become the continuous perceptual moment.

3) Retinally emitted spike fixed times over neural distance, acquire intrinsic latency, without latency coding, creating a lasting, spatially stable perceptual context that is synchronous in the same z section, with the retinal sustained and repeated transient response to external edge information. This result is due to parsing generic unit-time into 1) the fixed time of retinal spike emission, 2) the latency that the same z spike acquires over neural distance, 3) the sequence of each emitted and latent z spike as spikes move and 4) the proximal-distal synchrony of identical 1D z spikes transiently present in each RF-aligned z section. If emitted rate adjusts for spike speed and distance between synapses, then proximal fixed emitted times remain fixed as synchronous z loci move during the perceptual moment.

4) While speed is a quality measured at high receptor grain or with local instruments, as a specific distance/time, with convergence of many receptors into large cortical RFs, this local quality acquires a global neurally synthesized context of actual and perceived temporal and spatial stability, which accrues with proportional increases in spike latency and neural distance to cortical perceptual areas. For vision, this internal transformation is consistent with the external decline of optic flow with the expansive spatial distance from the sensory surface of all egocentric observers, conferring a larger unitary wavelength (or redshift) on a larger spatial volume, consistent with the constant distance/time ratio c.

5) High local speed of bits, or spikes, is necessary to transmit high data rates. Here 1D spikes are moving z locations, which acquire proportionally increased latency with distance, in the equation c = wavelength * frequency, without streaming temporally coded spatial information at high speed to a decoder or reconstituted as a 2D image. Rather, specific emitted locations/times, or spikes moving at a repeatable speed, dimensionally reduce aligned synaptic RFs in serial 2D surfaces stimulated by external x-y information. This neural mechanism of serial 2D reduction by convergent 1D z spikes temporally synchronizes convergent reemitted perceptual contexts with the high spatial and temporal resolution of sensory spike emissions.

6) The convergence of proximal to distal 1D z spikes does not multiplex data, but is temporally synchronous, via the proportional increase in both distance and latency of reemitted z spikes. The reemitted response at mapped synapses to coincident identical spikes of whatever qualitative origin, causes a perceptually synchronized cortical sense of spatial and temporal stability in the stream of identical distally reemitted 1D z spikes. Because identical spikes are 1D z locations that move distally with an increased latent context, rather than constituting a defined latency code or a stream of temporally coded information that reconstitutes an image at IT cortical areas, the continuous timing of 1D z perception phase-locks at frequencies impedance matched with high spike rates generated by shifting RGCs at FEM frequencies during fixation.

7) X-y spatial input convergence on serial arrays of synapses that reemit 1D z spike outputs, is a geometric property that neurally converges moving z locations into perceptions, concepts, generalized re-

definitions and dimensional reductions that do not retain informational sensory detail. This is how distance/time, or locally defined spike speed, integrates with the distance, latency and synchronized spike frequency to aligned synapses arranged in serial arrays, to synthesize a longer context of a perceptually stable, enduring distance/time. This latent property of spatially and temporally convergent spikes at synapses, is basic to emergent properties of human reasoning.

Repetitive Synchrony in the Orthogonal Surfaces of the Cerebellum

The mechanism at the root of the increased dragonfly precision as it closes on a target, discussed in the last chapter, may be the same as the continuous increase in precision as a mammal reaches and finally grasps an object. The literature on the neurophysiology of reaching in 3D is fragmented and contradictory in some details, but is ripe for integration, by understanding how the repeated 2D surfaces arranged orthogonally in the cerebellum (CB) coordinate. However, we must start at the cerebellar periphery, in the spinal tract, where proprioceptive neurons (PNs) bifurcate, sending excitatory spikes up the spine to the lateral reticular nucleus (LRN), which inputs into the CB, and in the other branch down the spine to motor neurons (MNs), which excite muscles in the hand (*Fig. 5.1*).[356] Direct

---
[356] Pivetta, C., Esposito, M., Sigrist, M., Arber, S. (2014) Cell <u>156</u>:537.

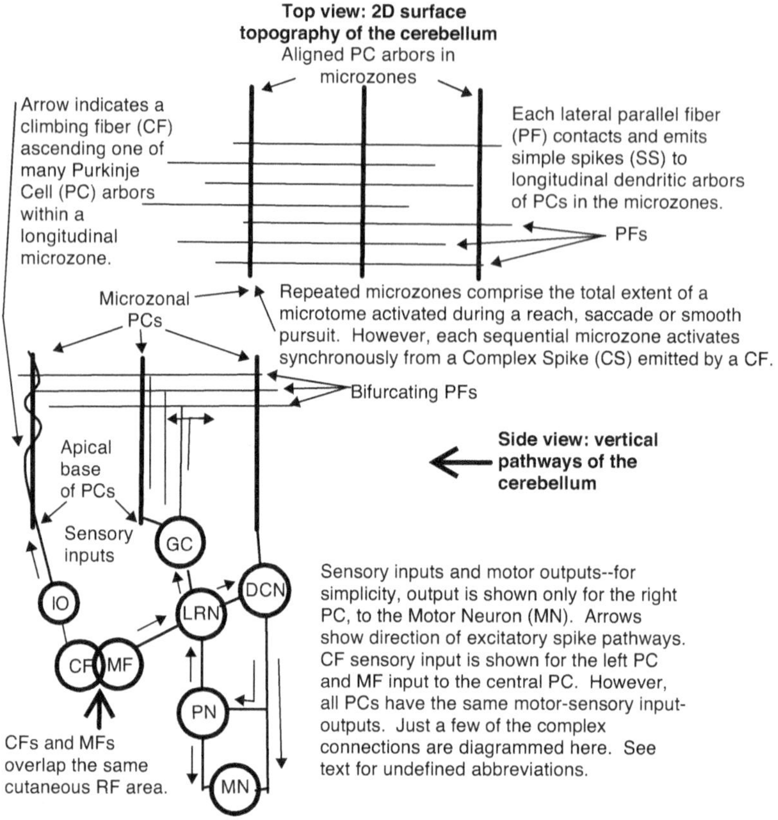

Top view: 2D surface topography of the cerebellum
Aligned PC arbors in microzones

Arrow indicates a climbing fiber (CF) ascending one of many Purkinje Cell (PC) arbors within a longitudinal microzone.

Each lateral parallel fiber (PF) contacts and emits simple spikes (SS) to longitudinal dendritic arbors of PCs in the microzones.

PFs

Microzonal PCs

Repeated microzones comprise the total extent of a microtome activated during a reach, saccade or smooth pursuit. However, each sequential microzone activates synchronously from a Complex Spike (CS) emitted by a CF.

Bifurcating PFs

Apical base of PCs

Side view: vertical pathways of the cerebellum

Sensory inputs

GC

IO

DCN

LRN

CF MF

PN

CFs and MFs overlap the same cutaneous RF area.

MN

Sensory inputs and motor outputs--for simplicity, output is shown only for the right PC, to the Motor Neuron (MN). Arrows show direction of excitatory spike pathways. CF sensory input is shown for the left PC and MF input to the central PC. However, all PCs have the same motor-sensory input-outputs. Just a few of the complex connections are diagrammed here. See text for undefined abbreviations.

Fig. 5.1: This scheme shows the cerebellum's repetitive structure (adapted from public sources and Azim et al., below).

excitatory efferent paths from cerebellar neurons to MNs are antecedent, which branch enroute to synapse at PNs; however, most of the input to PNs is inhibitory, from proprioceptive muscle spindle organs and other areas.[357] Selective ablation shows that the bidirectional PN pathway, which terminates at the same MN as the direct route, is necessary for quick, precise and accurate reaching and grasping by the hand.[358] In primates an additional direct

---

[357] Alstermark, B. & Isa, T. (2012) Ann. Rev. Neurosci. 35:559.

[358] Isa, T., Kinoshita, M. Nishimura, Y. (2013) Front. Neurol. 4:191; Azim, E., Fink, A., Jessell, T. (2014) Cold Spring Harbor Symp. Quant. Biol. 79:81; if the PN is inactivated, LRN-MN forelimb latency is much slower than the normal 3-5 msec; MN activity is also much reduced.

path from motor cortex to MNs has evolved, which bypasses the CB to increase the speed of practiced, highly coordinated movements, probably due to fewer synaptic delays.[359] Here, rather than forward prediction or negative feedback correction, excitatory and inhibitory inputs to the strategically positioned PNs are in a variable balance to increase or decrease the rate of excitatory output spikes.

Due to the PN bifurcation, identical z spikes split and move to distal LRN and MN x-y matched locations at the same time, roughly equal in distance. For invisible targets, visible feedback of spikes emitted by target locations to the SC and other retinotopic areas is replaced by proprioception from muscle spindles, which senses the degree of muscle contraction, but which is less accurate in gauging target location.[360] The flow of z spikes in opposite directions from the PNs must play a large role in the synchronous timing of cerebellar motor activity and motor activity in peripherally mapped limbs as they move.[361] This synchronous symmetrical precision is faster and of finer resolution than the latency of spikes in a spinal reflex arc to the fingers,[362] which is itself subliminally faster than the long neural

---

[359] Harel, R., Asher. I., Cohen, O., Israel, Z., Shalit, U., Yanai, Y., Zinger, N., Prut, Y. (2008) Behav. Brain Res. 194:119.

[360] Todorov, E. & Jordan, M. (2002) Nature Neurosci. 5:1226, say visual feedback is needed because occluding the subject's vision of the hand reaching toward a target increases positional variance; a visualized target here creates a long percept of foveal misalignment with the target. A subliminal motor map mismatch with the target at the SC is a quicker path requiring no long cortical perceptual time.

[361] Armstrong, D. & Edgely, S. (1984) J. Physiol. 352:403.

[362] Shadmehr, R., Smith, M., Krakauer, J. (2010) Ann. Rev. Neurosci. 33:89; they hypothesize that an efference copy to the CB accompanies the motor command, to predict motor target position, which is faster than a spinal reflex reacting to sensory information.

routes from sensory receptors to visual cortex as it perceives the hand and eye in unison.

Spinal interneurons fire at a faster rate within the long phase intervals of M1 cortical spike rhythms.[363] A MN does not fire unless its specific muscle is active, when the MN sustains fire at a high rate. This motor hierarchy of firing rates parallels the sensory hierarchy that sustains firing rates at small peripheral RFs; spatio/temporal convergence at successive synaptic levels, cause serial reductions in firing rate (*Fig. 5*). With fixed emitted times of spikes rather than a temporal code, high resolution of sensory and motor timing at the periphery requires high sustained rates if synchronized perceptually.

Here, the bifurcation at the PN is designed to match spikes at equally distant z locations at the same synchronous time at the same x-y mapped location, rather than to transfer information to a cerebellar location as an efference copy of a motor instruction, for predictive computation of a targeted goal.[364] PN emitted spikes also do not code feedback or feedforward data, but here are identical z locations that, since x-y is topographically identical at all levels, synchronize z time bidirectionally. Analytical sensory-motor distinctions are also not in 1D emitted PN spikes, which do not code divergent information to LRN and MNs. As part of slower M1 rhythms that synchronize with CB and MNs,[365] more repeti-

---

[363] Shalit, V., Zinger, N., Joshua, M., Prut, Y. (2012) Cereb. Cortex 22:1904.

[364] Azim, E. & Alstermark, B. (2015) Curr. Opin. Neurobiol. 33:16.

[365] Soteropoulos, D. & Baker, S. (2006) J. Neurophysiol. 95:1194; Hansen, S., Hansen, N., Christensen, L., Petersen, N., Nielsen, J. (2002) Exp. Br. Res. 146:282; Petersen, T., Willensley-Olsen, M., Conway, B., Nielsen, J. (2012) J. Physiol. 590:2443; Isa et al., op. cit.

tive peripheral spikes at 2D surfaces synchronize RF locations with delayed cortical perceptions (in *Fig. 4.2*). High rates of identical z spikes do not transfer data, only repetitive emitted times, necessary for synchronized precision between M1 and MNs.[366]

In the cerebellar cortex, a series of 'microzones' sequentially activate during a reaching action (*Fig. 5.1*). The thin microzone is made up of aligned cells and their dendritic arbors arranged end-to-end.[367] To presage coming detailed arguments, the microzone is a 2D surface, similar to the SC, so is a timing reference for a brief window of sensory input time. As one reaches toward a goal, the stages of movement progress, with new sensory input at each microzone; this on-the-fly input enables a quick response[368] while trajectory error is small and incipient. This repetitive mechanism prevents the accumulation of error to large amplitudes during a reach to a target, which would occur in a pre-programmed predictive path integrated over a total reach time that lasts a half-second or more.

A review of CB anatomy relevant to spike synchrony is in order (*Fig. 5.1*). Mossy fibers (MFs) and climbing fibers (CFs) are afferents from the same peripheral RF of muscle and skin, which input to the same point on CB surface topography where parallel fibers (PFs) cross microzones. These repeated microzones are a sequential map of peripheral topography. A single CF branch circles around the axonal stalk of a microzonal Purkinje Cell (PC), then winds separately around each of the dendritic branches making up its

---

[366] Ushiyama, J. & Ushiba, J. (2013) Clin. Neurophys. 124:5.

[367] Sugihara, I., Lang, E., Llinas, R. (1993) J. Physiol. 470:243.

[368] Shadmehr et al, op. cit.

arbor. Up to 1000 PCs make up each microzone; each PC arbor is about 200 x 200 x 10 micrometers. The thin dimension of 3-19 dendritic arbors, or fans, make up the total width of the microzone.[369] The longitudinal microzones are repeatedly crossed by the laterally oriented fields of excitatory PFs which bifurcate across the cerebellar surface from granule cells (GCs), which in turn project upward from the terminus of the MFs.

Areas of PFs have patchy topographical boundaries; because these areas overlap in extent, they serve to bridge diffuse borders and the ipsilateral and contralateral sides of the CB, which has no midline like the hemispheres of the cerebral cortex. Although most PFs at a topographic x-y location originate from the same cutaneous area as CFs, MF spikes of different shapes, due to differing receptor types, impinge on microzonal PCs from a large variety of locations.[370] Each microzone acts as a temporal gate, so that like the tremor gating of successive spike emission times at the retina, labeled MFs not cutaneously mapped to each microzone can synchronize with cutaneously mapped MFs as sequential microzones activate during a motor movement.

Peripheral receptors stimulate MFs and the roughly-bounded PF patches on the CB surface sequentially as muscles move; the total CB area activated by a limb reach is called a myotome. As a lateral myotome activates, the orthogonal longitudinally ori-

---

[369] De Zeeuw, C., Hoebeek, F., Bosman,L., Schonewille, M., Witter, L., Koekkoek, S. (2011) Nature Rev. Neurosci. $\underline{12}$:327; Heck, D. (1999) Neurosci. Lett. $\underline{263}$:137.

[370] Schwarz, C., Walsh, J. (2001) J. Neurophys. $\underline{86}$:2489; Ito, M. (1984) The Cerebellum and Neural Control; van Kan, P. Gibson, A, Houk, J. (1993) J. Neurophysiol. $\underline{69}$:74.

ented microzones activate sequentially. Each myotome comprises inputs from the sequential RFs of cutaneous skin and muscles, from the upper arm to the fingers or from the upper leg to the toes,[371] or the course of a smooth eye movement or saccade. The myotome RFs, via the patchy interlace of PF fields crossing the repeated microzones, must coordinate muscle groups within the context of whole joint movement,[372] rather than specifically controlling individual muscles, to make reaching or walking movements seamlessly continuous across the cortical midline in any direction, but with a continuously variable and adaptable route over time.

All the PCs comprising an individual microzone fire synchronously in response to synchronized CF input from topographically organized gap-junction coupled cells in the inferior olive (IO) of the brain stem.[373] A CF fires at slow rates of 1-2 spikes/sec, reemitting in the PC a large complex spike (CS) with several spikelets attached, lasting about 10 msec. That the CF winds around each PC stalk and arbor, to exert a high-amplitude CS one or two times each second, suggests that CSs are necessary to periodically inhibit other PC inputs for a period lasting a few to a few hundred msec. The CS is variously thought to be an error or reset signal. This CS-induced pause also transiently stifles the PC inhibitory output to muscles at that microzone.

For expository simplicity the circuitry will not be detailed, but PCs inhibit the deep cerebellar nuclei

---

[371] Apps, R. & Garwicz, M. (2005) Nature Rev. Neurosci. 6:297.

[372] Pruszinski, J., Kurtzer, I., Nashed J., Omrani, M., Brouwer, B., Scott, S. (2011) Nature 478:387.

[373] Sugihara, I., Marshall, S., Lang, E. (2007) J. Comp. Neurol. 501:13.

(DCN), which directly excite interneurons of the spine. Interneurons branch to PNs and continue down to MNs. Variable inhibition at PNs and DCNs gates the excitation necessary for sequential muscular movement.

While a single PC fires CSs at 1-2 Hz, populations of microzonal PCs synchronize CSs at up to 10 Hz during locomotion.[374] In smooth pursuit, CS rates do not increase in response to the magnitude of error, but increase due to pursuit speed, so are not an error signal.[375] Similar to the inhibition of V1 response and perception during each saccade,[376] CS inhibition of PC activity allows new simple spikes (SS) from peripheral MFs to refresh each microzone without recurrent older SS, which would disrupt the current state of the reach trajectory. The continuous renewal of SS, in the patchy PFs that input into the upper PC arbors, bridge the modifying context as the movement executes.

The CF-activated synchronized 10 Hz firing of CSs in each orthogonal microzone, is repeated sequentially in successive microzones during activation of the whole microtome.[377] Muscle activation starts with a highly synchronized state in all the microzones of the microtome just as the reach begins; this may synchronize the ballistic trajectory and the perceived

---

[374] Ozden, I., Dombeck. D., Hoogland, T., Tank, D., Wang, S. (2012) PLoS One 7:e42650. This reference has an accessible supplemental movie showing the activation of microzonal PCs during locomotion.

[375] Dash, S., Catz, N., Dicke, P., Thier, P. (2010) Exp. Br. Res. 205:41.

[376] Bridgeman et al. (1975), Burr et al., Wurtz, op. cit. Chap. Three.

[377] De Gruijl, Hoogland, T., De Zeeuw, C. (2014) J. Neurosci. 34:8937; Ozden et al., op. cit. Synchronous CS coactivations in microzones have maximal amplitude about 15 msec preceding motor activity, which is the approximate conduction time to the MNs.

goal. After this initial synchrony, frequencies become broadly distributed (desynchronized) as muscles activate sequentially, with a final microtome synchrony when the reach ends, for example, at a food pellet.[378] Also consistent with this data, when a macaque arm is stabilized in a precision grip, spikes synchronize during the whole holding period at M1 cortex and at the output DCNs.[379]

Each PF fires SS at high spontaneous rates, over 50 up to 100-200 spikes/sec[380] depending on experimental conditions; the rate also increases somewhat during movement or sensory stimulation. The laterally-oriented PFs stimulate SS in the PC dendritic fans making up the orthogonal microzones. Since CSs fire at such a low rate, even with the low efficiency of SS transfer from PFs to PC dendrites, 90% of PC activity is due to SS.[381] Most PFs at the cerebellar surface have thin diameters and are unmyelinated, so do not move spikes rapidly,[382] despite rapid, precise limb movements. Because PFs bifurcate like a 'T' along the microtome's axis (*Fig. 5.1*), they must act like the previously described PN bifurcation, that is, to bilaterally increase the presence of moving SS along the typical 5-7 mm length of the PF. This length is equivalent to about a 10 msec interval between spikes and bridges several

---

[378] Heck et al., op. cit. Chap. Four; Groth, J. & Sahin, M. (2015) Front. System Neurosci. 9:98.

[379] Soteropoulos & Baker, op. cit.

[380] Person, A. & Raman, I. (2012) Front. Neural Circ. 6:97.

[381] Wise, A., Cerminara, N., Marple-Horvat, O., Apps, R. (2010) J. Physiol. 588:2373.

[382] Brown, M. & Ariel, M. (2009) J. Neurophys. 101:474; the deeper layer nearer the soma of PCs is more likely to have myelinated PFs, in Wyatt, K. Tanapat, P., Wang, S. (2005) Europ. J. Neurosci. 21:2285.

microzones.[383] Coincidentally, approximately 10 msec is the period of transient synchronization of individual muscles in synergistic groups.[384] During movement, coordinated biphasic activation-inhibition of agonist-antagonist muscle groups occurs in cycles of about 100 msec during sequential PC spike activity,[385] which is similar to the maximal amplitude of 10 Hz synchrony of populations of PCs in each microzone.[386]

M1 cortex activates approximately 90-120 msec prior to finger muscle activity; this is similar to the fastest muscle reaction time to visually perceived perturbation during a reach.[387] Subconscious correction of a perturbed reach takes a round trip minimum of 50-60 msec,[388] which suggests brainstem (reticular formation and SC) and CB involvement. A simple reflex path, without any brainstem circuitry, from muscle stretch organs to spine and back to muscles has a shorter roundtrip latency of

---

[383] Heck, D. & Sultan, F (2002) Human Mov. Sci. 21:411; Jacobson, G., Rokni, D., Yarom, Y. (2008) Trends Neurosci. 31:617; Garwicz, M. Jorntell, H., Ekerot, C. (1998) J. Physiol. 512 (Part 1): 277.

[384] Hansen, N., Hansen, S., Christensen, L., Petersen, N., Nielsen, J. (2001) J. Neurophys. 86:1266.

[385] Murphy, J., Mackay, W., Johnson, F. (1973) Brain Res. 55:263; Vallbo, A. & Wessberg, J. (1993) J. Physiol. 469:673; Park, S., Tara, E., Khodakhah, K. (2012) J. Neurophys. 107:2453; Jontell, H. & Ekarot, C. (2002) Neuron 34:797; this data is from primates.

[386] Ozden et al., op. cit.; Kistler, W., van Hemmen, J., de Zeeuw, C. (2000) Prog. Br. Res. 124:275 discuss 100 msec time windows.

[387] Moran, D. & Schwartz, A. (1999) J. Neurophys. 82:2676; Kurtzer, I. (2014) Front. Integr. Neurosci. 8:99 reviews the timing data listed.

[388] Brown, P., Farmer, S., Halliday, D., Marsden, J., Rosenberg, J. (1999) Brain 122:461; lag is derived from the slope of the phase curve. A rapid M1 path is part of this subliminal latency, in Pruszinski et al., op. cit., Nashed, J., Crevecoeur, F., Scott, S. (2014) J. Neurosci. 34:1769.

25-45 msec. One-way latency from peripheral CF RF to CB microzone has a similar duration; MFs from the same peripheral RF have even shorter 5-14 msec latencies, so can input to CB microzones quickly during adaptive, on-the-fly movements.[389]

The CS synchronization[390] in PC arbors clears recent SS, so that only new SS input via the approximately 170,000 PF synapses on each PC dendritic arbor.[391] Each PC responds to a short window of PF excitation, due to fast feedforward interneuronal inhibition that sharpens the PC SS output to a 1 msec timing precision,[392] as each microzone activates. Precisely timed MF SS also input at the axonal base of the PC,[393] which may be the source of high-frequency synchrony in PCs.[394] Successive waves of these dual-input MF SS transmit current emission times stimulated by rapidly changing input from the periphery, within the PF context of continuous limb

---

[389] Murphy et al., op. cit.

[390] Ozden, I., Sullivan, M., Lee, M., Wang S. (2009) J. Neurosci. 29:10463; about 90% of PCs in a microzone have cross-correlated CSs firing within a span of 4 msec.

[391] Napper, R. & Harvey, R. (1988) J. Comp. Neurol. 274:168; Mittmann, W., Koch, U., Hausser, M. (2005) J. Physiol. 563(Pt 2):369; Isope, P., Dieudonne, S., Barbour, B. (2002) NY Acad. Sci. 978:164; similar to PYCs in the hippocampus already discussed, the ability to summate within 1 msec propagates synchronous APs to other synapses while inhibiting asynchronous spikes for up to 30 msec. This short summation window preserves the precision of the emitted time micro-memory of spikes moving at relatively constant speed.

[392] Mittmann, W., Koch, U., Hauser, M. (2005) J. Physiol. 563 (Part 2):369.

[393] Isope, P. & Barbour, B. (2002) J. Neurosci. 22:4668; Walter, J., Dizon, M., Khodakhah, J. (2009) J. Neurosci. 29:8462; the MFs input to GCs, which then excite in apparently equal proportions both the axon at the base of the PC, and via PFs, the dendritic fan of the PC.

[394] Groth & Sahin, op. cit.

movement and on-the-fly adaptation. The sequential muscle movement requires no successive approximation to a previously defined, spatially static goal because a foveal target's x-y-z value is renewed with each 10 Hz microzone cycle. This process means that the path of a flyball is not precisely predicted ahead of time, or the terminus of a saccade precisely defined at initiation, but is approximate at low resolution. As the saccade or the reach toward a goal proceeds, serial microzones activate with more precise timing from SS inputs.

The greater precision with greater latency during the reach, saccade or smooth pursuit, is conventionally thought to be due to the increased effect of delayed negative feedback that takes over from the rapid ballistic feedforward process that presides at the beginning. Alternatively here, this increase in precision is contained in the shorter latencies of MF fixed emission-time spikes, in the most recently active microzones as the hand and/or the fovea nears the target. Also, MF inputs to PCs shift from a target's distant low 2D resolution to a high spike rate and resolution from looming receptors, emitted as sequential z locations/times, as the target nears.[395]

The interpretation here is that the bifurcations in PFs and at PNs pass twinned, synchronized z spikes to enable increasingly precise, serial 2D maps of emitted spike z locations of the positions of the target, hand and fovea. One must remember that because spikes here are emitted z times, not coded data, as distance shortens, spikes increase rate due to in-

---

[395] Popa, L., Streng, M., Hewitt, A., Ebner, T. (2015) Cerebellum online, p. 1; this shift to a velocity signal also occurs perceptually in optic flow; due to the effects of egocentric perspective, the stability of distant objects becomes a moving local speed, because the object has greater temporal and spatial resolution close to the observer.

creased stimulus motion near the receptor: frequency (or spike rate) = a constant average spike speed/wavelength (or target distance). Corrective shifts due to small deviations of the target on an x-y surface like the SC (discussed in Chapter Three), or at terminal microzonal surfaces as a target looms closer, can happen without consciously perceived intervention, or with the conventional necessity for long predictive computations or of looping negative feedback. The sequence of active x-y microzones and progression on the myotome z axis, defines only the next MF-active increment toward an M1 cortical goal-plan defined by a long-term M1 memory. The sequence of readjusting x-y target locations as the fovea follows the target, synchronized with the sequence of microzonal activations via PNs, explains how reaching motions to the same goal can have different paths and speeds, yet with the same precise endpoint.[396]

The continuous variation in muscle activity in the course of on-the-fly adaptations has been studied in macaques, with repeated trials in the smooth pursuit of a target. In this experiment, PC spike rates in the floccular region of the CB, together with behavioral measures of the pursuit, that is, the position, speed and acceleration of the fovea as it tracked the target, were recorded in the same trial. The trials were pooled and data aggregated into mean values; individual trial-to-trial variation, of spike rates correlated with the above behavioral measures, were also graphed.[397] An equation converted the average behaviorial measures described

---

[396] Morasso, P. (1981) Exp. Br. Res. 42:223.

[397] Medina, J. & Lisberger, S. (2007) J. Neurosci. 27:6832; Chaisenguanthum, K., Joshua, M., Medina, J., Binen, W., Lisberger, S. (2014) eNeuro 1:ENEURO 0004-14.2014.

above, to a single dimension of average firing rate in a single PC.[398] This regression model was found to successfully predict spike rates for the input behavioral motor responses, when compared with the actual values measured from the PC in a single trial. Usually this information is lost, because in an attempt to get a reliable signal without the variable spike rates in individual neurons, trial data is pooled.[399] But the individual variance recorded on each trial, of increased spike rates at smooth pursuit initiation (at least 100 msec after the target starts moving) and for the following 100 msec (following the schema in *Fig. 3.1*), were found to correlate highly with the variance of the behavioral measures for that trial. In other words, when smooth pursuit initiates, a specific behavior, such as the differing initiation time, correlates with the emission time of a specific spike in a PC.

This high timing correlation in a specific PC was found to decline over the steady-state pursuit that lasted over a half-second. One might expect successive activation of PCs as smooth pursuit progresses would decrease correlated precision at the same continuously recorded PC. Also, a transient high spike rate may correlate with initial pursuit because the same PC neurons are responding to the

---

[398] Conventionally, this 1D firing rate is a reduction in information content from the inputs. But since identical spikes here are instants of emitted time and location that converge synchronously at synapses, no image information is coded. More relevant, is the synchronization over z distance in *Fig. 4.4*, at sequential synapses in 2D arrays (*Fig. 3.4*), rather than sequential transmission of temporally coded sparse information.

[399] To increase reproducibility, large numbers of trials are necessary to reduce individual trial variability (Button, K., Ioannidis, J., Mokrysz, C., Nosek, B., Flint, J., Robinson, E., Munafo, M. (2013) Nature Rev. Neurosci. 14:365). However, with noisy variables controlled, greater precision is possible if a single trial is not averaged with other trials.

transitions from the same foveal fixation site, even though target initiation times and directions are randomized with each trial. During the steady-state after pursuit initiates, the sequential activation of microzones and muscles causes correlated changes in spike rates at distributed electrode locations, as well as of transiently synchronized average frequencies (if also recorded).

Despite the correlation of high spike rates recorded at local cells with a specific phase of a slow theta rhythm, spike rates like those in individual V1 cells discussed in Chapter Three, are not directly convertible to frequency recorded from large groups of neurons averaged over time and cortical area from a repeated stimulatory event.[400] This could result because spike rate after an initial event diminishes, or may vary with distance from the recording electrode; whereas synchrony is a statistical average of repeated spikes in the same neurons recorded in bins aggregated over time at each electrode. While distributed PC rhythms at up to 10 Hz are recorded during locomotion,[401] local PC groups synchronize at over 200 Hz, due to recurrent connections with nearby PCs. This synchronous pooled measurement is much higher in frequency than spike rates of single PCs in the same population.[402] Average axonal spike speeds and synaptic summation times affect

---

[400] Panzeri et al. op. cit. Chap. Four; individual latencies were measured in 100 barrel column cells to the same repeated stimulus of an aligned whisker; almost all had the same (synchronous) 10-15 msec latency. However, spike rates pooled in sequential 5 msec bins in all the D2 barrel cells, to the same stimulus, were less precise over time.

[401] Ozden et al., op. cit.; as also stated, single PCs fire at 1-2 Hz spike rates at rest.

[402] de Solages, C., Szapiro, G., Brunel, N., Hakim, V. Isope, P. Buisseret, P., Rousseau, C., Barbour, B., Lema, C. (2008) Neuron 58:775.

the phase-locked timing between the synchronized cell groups, in which spike temporal intervals and velocities synchronize and integrate as a single z time dimension at the specific distances and latencies between the recording electrodes.

In contrast to smooth pursuit, a saccade is analyzed in a cell population in the following experiment,[403] because two PC types, 'bursters' and 'pausers', are active at the same time. Aggregate SS rates are pooled from these cells recorded one cell at a time, over repeated trials. These pooled PC responses from the posterior vermis of the CB, show an increase in rate with the combined increase in speed and associated magnitude of the saccade.[404]

To summarize the data, in pausers, a mean spike rate of about 100 SS/sec abruptly reduces by more than half, thereby disinhibiting the saccade as its trajectory starts; bursters progressively increase mean rate to about 75 SS/sec from saccade start till saccade end; the latter rate then decreases to a few spikes/sec, the baseline level, while pausers resume their previous high rate. A saccade as short as 38 msec in duration, sustains 100 msec of aggregate PC activity, perhaps to sustain downstream convergent activity. The population data shows that a balance in peak spike rates, of necessarily equal numbers of bursters and pausers, determines the combined speed and length of the saccade. The pausers and bursters converge in a 50:1 ratio on cell clusters

---

[403] Herzfeld, D., Kojima, Y., Soetedjo, R., Shadmehr, R. (2015) Nature 526:439; of course, with variable responses in individual PCs with repeated trials, these average spike rates are not valid for any specific PC at any specific time.

[404] Speed and distance of the saccade are integrated as one spike rate. Due to the 1D limitations of spike rate, to increase the magnitude of the saccade, the speed of the saccade also has to increase.

in the caudal fastigial nucleus. A cluster's summated output inputs to oculomotor neurons that control eyeball movement discussed in Chapter Three, in which aggregate spike rate controls a saccade's combined speed and magnitude.

Within the CB, experimenter-defined 'error corrective feedback' and 'feedforward prediction' are indicated by temporary increases in spike rate, but both signals are found in the same neuron, which is too low in the hierarchy of neural assemblies to 'understand' or cognitively process the (presumed) difference in temporal codes. In the following study,[405] 72% of PCs recorded had a temporally shifted increase in spike rate that averaged 223 msec before and a lagging increase in spike rate that averaged 227 msec after, the PC spikes continuously recorded as the fovea followed and the hand reached toward an unpredictably moving target.

These increases in spike rates in single PCs at approximately equal lead and lag times (with wide 130-150 msec ranges) are calculated from regression equations of the same form as those in the Medina & Lisberger smooth pursuit experiment described earlier. These transiently high spike rates could be mistaken for predictive long cerebellar computations, via neural loops of feedback information, that refine the motor route to the target over time. Conventionally the presumption is that the high PC spike rate that leads and lags the motion, increases encoded information about positive feedforward and negative feedback error. The delayed increase in spike rate increases proportionally to the error, perhaps due to increased sensory inputs delayed through multiple synapses, from long-latency

---

[405] Popa, L., Hewitt, A., Ebner, T. (2012) J. Neurosci. 32:15345.

visual perception and cognitive assessment of the proximity of the hand to the target. This sensory-motor mismatch at 2D surfaces, such as at the SC and serially in the CB, may correct small errors subliminally as they occur, but also requires cognitive and perceptual latencies of about 250 msec that assess larger errors as they change over time.

Early in the reach trajectory in the above experiment, the temporarily high PC spike rate due to perceived error appears first, then during steady-state the forward prediction signal appears also, so is a bimodal signal. The late reach trajectory keeps only the transient forward predictive high spike rate as the goal is reached.[406] This predictive PC spike rate stays present as the x-y position signal shifts to a local speed signal in proximity to the goal. However, this predictive signal does not shorten in latency as the goal nears. This is a clue that the predictive advance in PC spike rate is not encoding motor information of increasing accuracy in spikes; higher spike rates have shorter intervals, therefore precision, synchronized though delayed from cortical associative and perceiving areas. As discussed in Chapter Two, a predictive forward plan is equivalent to, and based on, recycled memory; bimodal timing symmetries of increased spike rates are expressions of this ultimate z equivalence in neurons.

Conventionally, both long-distance prediction and multi-joint coordination, require computation with defined reference coordinates over a whole reach trajectory, with changes in each muscle over the temporal sequence, aggregating and changing as the movement unfolds, along with delayed feedback, a calculation that taxes the ability of modern

---

[406] Popa, Streng et al. op. cit.

computers.[407] But here, repetitive circuits in each microzone use newly emitted MF spikes, x-y aligned topography and synchronous-sequential time shown in *Figs. 4.2-4.4*, to avoid the computation of complex muscle and joint dynamics from stable reference points. The short-latency MF inputs to PFs provide successive contexts to PC arbors as microzones sequentially activate. Also, the temporally precise PC SS outputs topographically synchronize, in successive microzones, sensory LRN input and MN output, via twin spikes that split bilaterally from each spike that inputs to PNs. This serially renewed synchrony adjusts to reaching inaccuracies just-in-time as the target nears, without long neural routes from negative feedback loops. Here, dimensional reduction of repeated microzonal x-y surfaces to a dynamic 3D structure is via z spike synchrony.

A slow synchronized frequency of 1.5-2.5 Hz prevails over the cortical motor areas, DCNs and the CB.[408] To the experimenter, these are plans, or predictions, of future motor actions based on past learned behaviors. But to a spike, a long interval makes static the fixed-time of spike emission, a fixed plan translocated over long neural distances within the same topographically mapped circuitry. Slow synchronous rhythms result from fixed-emission times, or spike micro-memories, from serially reemitted sequentially active inputs from relevant brain areas into a phase-locked order.

---

[407] Scott, S. (2004) Nature Rev. Neurosci. 5:532.

[408] Shalit et al., op. cit.; a resting M1 rate of 15 spikes/sec ramps up to about 30 spikes/sec as the reach starts, but then declines back to the resting rate during a maintained grasp, while spinal neurons downstream have ramped up from 25 spikes/sec to a maintained rate of about 40 spikes/sec for the duration of the grasp. Rowland, N., Goldberg, J., Jaeger, D. (2010) Neurosci. 166:698 describe these slow synchronized rhythms in more detail.

Transient local synchronous frequencies must characterize continuous muscle movement, but may be hard to analyze at high resolution with frequencies averaged over many trials on the M1 surface. As stated a few paragraphs ago, the stationary state just before and at the terminus of a reach creates synchrony in the whole microtome. Synchrony is not only an indication of precision over x-y aligned neural z distance while spikes are present at the same time and locations, but indicates, by pooled phase-locking, redundant information that is not changing, and therefore is not transmitted.[409] Here, peripheral information, transduced at receptors as emitted-time micro-memory spikes, remains spatially and temporally precise at the periphery. Synchronization between the periphery and cortical areas, of moving 1D z spikes transiently present at aligned RFs in 2D surfaces, does not move information as phase differentials at stationary electrodes recording average frequencies, but here reduces repeated 2D surfaces to a sequence of x-y-z resonances. RF-aligned 1D z spikes at a resonant frequency dissolve spatial and temporal gaps between specific 2D surfaces, whether in the CB, the serial stages of vision or other sensory systems.

Locally transient synchronized frequencies lose precision in the statistically averaged synchronization recorded from populations of spikes at a static location, as occurs in the pooling of trials and spikes, already described. That SS in the same PC neuron are +225 and -227 msec signals, and also respond to all the behavioral motor measures of the reach

---

[409] Mizuseki & Buzsaki, op. cit. Chap. Four; Pitkow, X., Liu, S., Angelaki, D., DeAngelis, G., Pouget, A. (2015) Neuron $\underline{87}$:411; the latter argue that single neurons correlate better with behavioral thresholds than pooled correlations because pooled redundancy is associated with limited information.

(its speed, direction and distance), shows that one neuron does not integrate multiplexed information, but responds indiscriminately to convergent 1D z spike inputs[410] with varying spike times. The re-emitted spike rate in individual neurons has to vary with emitted times that synchronously converge in least-time. Proximally sustained, identical 1D z spikes here do not encode conventional information, but reemit to synchronize the high resolution and dimensionality of emitted spikes with distal cognitive and perceptual convergent z latencies (*Fig. 4.6*). Averaging cortical spike frequencies over time shows this filtered synchronization at specific electrode locations, but averaging also reduces the resolution of spike timing on specific neural routes. The best current explanation is that this "heterogeneous mixture of selectivity" is a population code.[411] As with spatial frequency coding and univariant somatosensory responses discussed earlier,[412] overlapping responses in populations of neurons constitute impedance matching, in that activity in cortical cells may shift over time, but reliably reemit a latent perception from a stimulus input range in labeled neurons.

One can argue that high sustained gamma frequencies that range to slower theta and alpha rhythms over larger cortical expanses, constitute a scale-free power law.[413] Most studies that measure averaged frequencies filter out arrhythmic spikes by subtract-

---

[410] Prince et al., op. cit. Chap. Three; Popa, Hewitt et al. op. cit.

[411] Panzeri, S., Macke, J., Gross, J., Kayser, C. (2015) Trends Cogn. Sci. $\underline{19}$:162.

[412] De Valois et al., op. cit. Chap. One, Harvey et al., op. cit. Chap. Four.

[413] He, B., Zempel, J., Snyder, A., Raichle, M. (2010) Neuron $\underline{66}$:353; this population code is here interpreted to be a univariant response.

ing noise to a pre-stimulus baseline. He et al. find that this arrhythmic noise is not due to transient signals of varying frequencies and amplitudes averaged over time, and is not due to instrumentally introduced noise. They find that a persisting arrhythmia depends on the location of the electrode on the cortical surface; this local arrhythmia becomes a specific synchronized frequency only with the onset of specific types of motor activity. This synchronization indicates fixational perception of the specific motor activity as it occurs (*Figs. 4.2, 4.4*).

Past references show that sustained high rates in proximal neurons, fire within a specific phase of slower cortical rhythms.[414] Peripheral emitted spike frequencies and gamma rhythms, synchronous at V1 level and other cortical areas, likewise integrate into specific phases of slow theta rhythms.[415] The local neurons recorded at a cortical electrode also synchronize different spike rates at consistently differing phase times of two or more divergent frequencies.[416] This may be a measure of precision, or a distributed response among many neurons that becomes perceived as precision, if reemitted from convergent synchronized inputs into long-latency perception (*Fig. 4.6*). As already stated, emitted-time precision is lost if statistical pooling is used to reduce the noise in individual neuronal responses. What is construed as desynchronization when signals recorded at a static electrode are pooled, are actually temporarily precise synchronizations at

---

[414] Montemurro et al., op. cit.

[415] Canolty et al., op. cit.

[416] Phase-locking in a single neuron can occur at different spike rates at different phases of the same frequency, in Jacobs J., Kahana, M., Ekstrom, A., Fried, I. (2007) J. Neurosci. 27:3839.

shifting locations near the electrode. The experimenter, by controlling the variability of continuous stimulation to ensure repeatability of standardized stimuli, also reduces the precision of any specific recorded response.[417]

Not only are one or two least-time z spikes necessary in IT cells for object identification,[418] but in recent experiments using Principal Components Analysis (PCA) to reduce the many dimensions of the population responses of IT cells, results show that individual IT cells respond preferentially to one dimension (or facial feature),[419] reemitting as stated here, to the anatomical convergence of temporally synchronous spikes. The spatial pattern of the overlapping responses of ~205 IT cells were separated by the PCA method into 25 appearance and 25 shape features that identified specific faces. 68% of the variance in spike rate was predictive of a specific appearance feature, as measured in a late-stage Anterior Medial (AM) IT cell. The 1D feature selectivity in an AM cell was shown as a maximal spike rate with greatest stimulus intensity, firing at linearly lower rates to similar appearance features; but an AM cell's higher spike rate was orthogonally invari-

---

[417] Panzeri et al., op.cit. Chap. Four.

[418] Hung et al., op. cit. Chap. Three, find highest object categorization and identification rates in the initial 12.5 msec window in the average range of 110-150 msec latencies for spikes to arrive at IT cells after retinal stimulation. In their experimental design, the recording bin for analysis expanded from 12.5 msec to 200 msec. Sugase et al., op. cit. Chap. Three, recorded the highest spike rates, within a 50 msec sliding bin, at about 110 msec after stimulus onset. The results show that high firing rate corresponds with higher psychophysical precision over an approximate 110-150 msec latency range. Here, stimulation to the length of the fixation period allows proximal spatial-temporal resolution to synchronize with perceptual spikes in distal cortex.

[419] Chang, L. & Tsao, D. (2017) Cell 169:1013, stimuli were presented for 150 msec, bin sizes ranging over 50-300 msec.

ant not only to facial orientation, but to all the other feature dimensions of a specific face. It is argued that the high spike rate to one feature is greater information, but the investigators also admit that how spike activity encodes information is unknown.[420] Here, emitted spikes spatially and temporally summate rapidly at selective cortical synapses, so re-emit higher rates as higher perceptual intensity and resolution. That the same AM cell responds at highest rate to one feature dimension in closely timed trials agrees with the notion that the most rapid 1D z spikes in multiple IT cells synchronize with retinal 2D information during the fixation period (*Fig. 4.5*).

Noisy signals may converge to synchronize at the dendritic fields of locally grouped neurons, such as the typical 50-100 cells in a cortical column. Hypothetically, if inputs of 100 spikes/sec from multiple cortical neurons impinge on a dendritic arbor within a short temporal window, this will cause reemitted output in that cortical level at the same rate.[421] But the variable spike output intervals and rates in any single neuron,[422] mean that a precise emitted-time is perceived only if reemitted spikes in a cortical population temporally synchronize with labeled RGC inputs and endures in a perceptual moment (*Fig. 4.2*). The experimenter may interpret the unknown origins or emission times of individual cortical spikes as 'noise' because the electrode is not sited at the right location in the proper time window. However, the idea that spikes have no explicitly coded information, but rather are fixed emission times, is more

---

[420] Meyers, E., Borzello, M., Freiwald, W., Tsao, D. (2015) J. Neurosci. 35:7069.

[421] Shadlen, M. & Newsome, W. (1998) J. Neurosci. 18:3870.

[422] Jacobs et al., op. cit.

relevant to the variable timing of 1D spike inputs and outputs at any linked synapse.

Higher proximal spike rates from higher stimulus intensities input into larger cortical RFs, to not only synchronize proximal resolution with perceived intensity, but greater summation and reemission speed from convergence (this includes the higher PC spike rates at -227 msec that increase with the degree of visually perceived error).[423] The x-y misalignments of forward predictive (ballistic) and presumed negative feedback signals for the late trajectories of saccades, smooth pursuits and reaches, associated with higher spike rates, increase the re-emitted least-time precision of muscles in the sequence of microzones activated in the whole microtome. Synchronization occurs rapidly in M1 cells at relatively high frequency at the beginning of a reach, but at low spike rates.[424] Here, low spike rates in M1 cells increase intervals to stabilize a plan of motor activity so that a micro-memory is fixed over neural distance. The same cells do not have high spike rates until the reach is well underway, which is perhaps necessary to activate larger muscles rapidly via convergence and in the late trajectory, to increase spatial and temporal precision. The rapid M1 synchronization at low spike rate indicates, similarly to the Maldonado et al. results discussed in the last chapter, a synthesis of multiple 2D surfaces at any fixed time as one 2D surface (*Fig.3.4*), rather than slower information transfer over time.

---

[423] Perceived mismatch error in a previously known sequence creates a generic increase in spike rate in hippocampal areas, as compared to an unpredictable or novel stimulus; in Garrido, M., Barnes, G., Kumaran, D., Maguire, E., Dolan, R. (2015) Neuroimage 120:362.

[424] Hatsopoulos, N., Ojakangas, C., Paninski, L., Donaghue, J. (1998) PNAS (USA) 95:15706; synchrony and spike rate are both dependent on the direction-of-trajectory selectivity of the M1 cell.

Previous references have described a combined ballistic feedforward and negative feedback that control movements, though there is little evidence that the CB calculates long-range trajectories from internal reference coordinates. There are also suggestions in the literature that conventional ballistic feedforward and negative feedbacks are shared over rapid and delayed time scales, here synchronized as a constant distance/time ratio on a 1D z axis, in which sensory-motor information loses its separate distinctions, to manifest phenomenologically and perceptually, as real-time error correction.[425] Consistent with studies already described, individual, not pooled trials explicitly show this increased prediction accuracy with increased latency after a reach perturbation, because the x-y alignments and higher spike rates allow least-time reemitted z timing accuracy to inhibit slower inputs rather than be conmingled as averaged, pooled data with large standard deviations, confidence intervals or error bars. Here, one can dispense with the engineering abstractions of delayed negative and predictive positive feedback, or the analytical distinction between sensory and motor spikes (imposed on identical 1D bidirectional PN spikes) that synchronize LRN with MNs. *Figs. 4.2, 4.4 and 4.5,* derived from other evidence, integrate these proximal rapid and distal delayed time scales into a 1D z time diagram superimposed on orthogonal serial x-y surfaces. These identical 1D spikes have precise emitted times and latencies which serially filter to the longer latencies and intervals of perceptual spikes, seen in the synchronous time of a z section. The cortical perception of target-foveal map error, also summates and synchronizes more spikes rapidly with peripheral motor

---

[425] Wagner, M. & Smith, M. (2008) J. Neurosci 28:10663.

neurons to correct via least-time inhibition of slower, less accurate inputs.

The delay (of closed loop negative feedback) that makes motor prediction increasingly accurate in reaching, saccade or smooth pursuit experiments by applying the same algorithm repeatedly, is here required so that sustained 1D z spikes (here with no coded, tagged or labeled information) input at serial orthogonal layers of synapses, to reemit, from synchronous inputs, as delayed perception. Contrary to the idea that spikes economically encode information in the subliminal CB, PC spikes sustain for 100 msec after a short 38 msec saccade;[426] this long period may be required to synchronize spikes in proximal MNs and receptors with distal latent percepts in visual and motor cortical areas. To generalize: the longer the neural distance between the receptor type and the labeled perceptual area, the longer the sustained receptor response lasts (such as by FEM-generated RGC spikes during fixation) so that the proximal receptor and distal perceptual area have temporally synchronous edge-specific spikes (*Fig. 4.4*). Spike synchrony is necessary for proximal-distal 'division of labor', defined earlier, which allows a convergent perception to RF-align with proximally sustained, temporally and spatially precise inputs.

Repeated 2D synaptic arrays filter x-y alignment errors by least-time competition between peripheral (RGC or MF) RFs and latent, distal (cortical or microtomal) RFs. What in engineering terms is a 'state predictor' based on an initial synchronized state at the start of a trajectory, orients newly emitted z spikes at the terminus of the trajectory, into the

---

[426] Herzfeld et al., op. cit.

synchronized topographically mapped M1 fixed-time plan, or memory, of reduced rate latent spikes. This process occurs in the same z section (the synchronous time state in *Figs. 4.2, 4.4, 4.6*), so that perceived error, where target z spikes are located on a sensory x-y surface, converges least-time routes of the planned x-y motor end-point with the z spikes generated at the present x-y target location.

The synchrony of identical 1D spikes between serially aligned RFs on topographic maps correlates long duration, long interval, perhaps imprecise convergent perceptual z spikes with sustained, newly emitted spikes that have high temporal and spatial resolution at a proximal sensor array. An initial spike response moves at a consistent speed and with a synchronously emitted time, to the first cortical synapse, as detailed for whisker stimulation in rodents and vision in turtle retina RGCs.[427] It is this peripheral x-y spike precision and reliability that synchronizes with delayed perception, which 'binds' the summation of near-synchronous inputs at serially convergent synapses with the external objective event that generated the least-time emitted times of z spikes. Emitted time, not a derived temporal code, is an intrinsically precise property of the 1D z spike, as discussed for the initiation of smooth pursuit,[428] shown also in *Figs. 4.1* and *4.2*. This fixed emitted time is due to the x-y synchrony of FEM-stimulated spikes at an initial 2D surface; equal latencies of z spikes at maximally responsive summat-

---

[427] Panzeri et al., op. cit., Chap. Four; Greschner et al., op. cit. Chap. One.

[428] Medina & Lisberger, Chaisenguanthum et al., op. cit.; Osborne, Hohl et al., op. cit. Chap. Three, show a timing threshold graph that has no standard deviations, or error, for the initiation of pursuit, demonstrating that a precise fixed time initiates as z spikes start to move.

ing synapses in serial 2D arrays rapidly reemit. The temporal and spatial summations that accrue over neural distance in serially convergent 2D arrays increase the synchronized perception of temporal stability due not only to longer intervals between z spikes, but identical emitted z times in the same sequential instant of synchronous time (*Fig. 4.4*). Labeled serially connected RFs repeat retinotopy but reemit z spikes, which are the perceived, continuously enduring dimension, not a hypothetical reconstituted stable x-y image in distal cortex.

One should compare a current method for reducing the dimensions of experimental brain data with the reduction of 2D surfaces by synchronous convergent 1D z spikes as demonstrated here. This other method adapts a version of PCA to reduce the dimensions of a reaching movement recorded by an electrode array on the surface of motor cortex of primates.[429] The rhythmic changes in firing rates of many neurons are smoothed and averaged for the analysis of a movement over time. This method captures 50-70% of the variance in the data, as the reaching movement traverses various routes and different neurons over aggregate time to the same endpoint. Unless a reference synaptic array synchronizes spike output, it is unknown with this methodology where and when spikes at a cortical electrode array originate, so this and other heterogeneous properties characterize much of the data variance. By aggregating heterogeneous data for population analysis, noisy single neuron data is lost in favor of statistically tractable pooling. But similar

---

[429] Churchland, M., Cunningham, M., Kaufman, M., Foster, J., Nuvujukian, P., Ryu, S., Shenoy, K. (2012) Nature 487:51; Shenoy, K., Kaufman, M., Sahani, M., Churchland M. (2011) Prog. Br. Res. 192:331; descriptions and videos show the rotation of the movement in time, but not in distance, as projected on a 2D state space.

to experiments described earlier, pooled data can be separated into single trials, which is more predictive of the reduced variation (e.g. of reaction time) in the next trial.

This analysis of magnitude and duration of population responses measured with electrode arrays on motor and premotor cortex, in the preparation for a reach, shows 'condition invariance', that is, spike rates do not vary with behavioral direction, speed or distance; but reaction time changes rates and durations, orthogonal to the invariant conditions.[430] This relates to the theory here that spikes are not an informational temporal code but are 1D z locations and times that temporally synchronize proximally-distally. *Figs. 4.2-4.6* show how sustained emitted times of spikes synchronize precisely, without averaging spike rates at electrodes over time. If serial electrode arrays were to map adapting neuronal routes with locations of proximal spikes that distally reemit, the varying population responses that are part of decoder algorithm designs, would have more precision, therefore more predictive value.

With the proper assumptions about the behavior of spikes, neurons and synapses, one can not only arrive at conclusions that reduce the high-dimensional amalgam of spike data, but create a testable template that formalizes brain mechanisms. At present metadata seeks to integrate the results of various experiments, via standardization that use one metric to dissolve differences in techniques and methodologies. As discussed in the last two paragraphs, variability and large deviations in aggregate data can be more precise if reduced to individual trials,

---

[430] Kaufman, M., Seely, J., Sussillo, D., Ryu, S., Shenoy, K. Churchland, M. (2016) eNeuro 3:0085-16.

and by extension, to moving spike locations mapped between specific emitting and remitting locations. High dimensional data pooled over time requires reductive techniques to perhaps resolve causal relationships, while the analysis here synchronizes RF-aligned locations of emitted and latent z spikes at precise times (*Fig. 4.4*). Otherwise a standardization based on assumptions convenient for experimentation, increases complexity and less understanding of the actual mechanisms at play.

For one interconnected hypothesis developed here, this means that for the overlap of retinal tremor frequency and gamma frequency in V1 at approximately 80 Hz, correctly positioned electrodes will record z synchronization between serial x-y locations that jibe exactly with emitted times, synaptic summation times and total latency of the neural pathway between the two locations. Earlier evidence in RGC, LGN, cerebellum and hippocampus, described synchronous input spikes that reemit with a 1 msec precision. Unless the brain perceives slow rhythms as collective averages over time measured from adjacent synapses, temporal precision of serially synchronized z spikes (*Figs.4.2, 4.4*), rather than a pooled average, is necessary for the brain's function at any point in time and should be definable with evolving experimental methodology.

The global perception of external image stability, here is a result of spatially and temporally synchronized spikes at 2D surfaces that reemit due to gamma synchrony. As discussed, this synchronization may be due to synergy of mistimed spikes at convergent synapses that summate to mass action for an aggregate, reemitted accuracy. Synchronization may also result from recurrent inhibition by convergent perception that selects least-time aligned inputs.[431] What is measured as an average gamma frequency is interpreted here to be precise synchronies of specific spike pairs emitted between connected synapses. Here intervals between repeated spikes, coupled with a constant spike speed, transiently synchronize at specific distances connecting synapses in serial 2D surfaces. The reduced frequency that is measured with increased neural distance and spike latency, is temporally and energetically more efficient than the actual transfer of peripheral information, imbedded in the fixed emitted times of identical z spikes. Rather than transferring massive information over neural distance to be decoded in cortex, or averaging collective 1D spikes to get a repeatable signal, individual neurons synchronize sustained 1D z spike intervals or rates to integrate proximal and distal synaptic locations in the same perceptual moment, as shown in *Fig 4.2*.

Because the minimum fixation duration of 150 msec is approximately the minimal length of the perceptual moment described in Chapter Three, the fastest identical spikes from object edges have endured convergent stages from the periphery, to excite IT cortical 1D spikes at serially synchronous times. *Figs. 4.4-4.5* show that the establishment of synchronies in parallel z sections, in spikes that have intrinsic properties of emitted time, latency, synchrony and location, enables transiently precise temporal synchronies. Timing precision is necessary in the CB, to synchronize motor response with new spikes stimulated by receptors as a reach nears a target. This process requires synchronized instants

---

[431] Litwin-Kumar, A., Rosenbaum, R., Doiron, B. (2016) J. Neurophys. $\underline{115}$:1399; several types of inhibitory neurons stabilize neural network responses in mouse V1 simulations. Here visual image stability may result via the recurrent inhibition necessary to synchronize tremor-generated spikes with V1 gamma frequencies.

of the same emitted time (*Fig. 4.4*), so that the least-time latency at a distal perceptual surface converges x-y mapping errors toward a perceptually synchronous target. What is a distally static target acquires flow, or speed, as it nears and moves past each receptor in a 2D array, stimulating a more precise spatial and temporal sense via higher spike rates. Serially reduced spike rates divide proximal-distal labor without moving or multiplexing high dimensional information to cortex for latent feedback.

In contrast to the sensory-motor synchronization of repeated 2D surfaces with sustained spikes stimulated by peripheral information, tactile and visual sensors used in current robot grasping technology have less temporal resolution nearer the target due to faster optical flow, which overloads algorithms with the data rates of changing target position.[432] MHz sensor data rates may be orders of magnitude higher than spike rates, but this is not only excessive information in each image frame reconstructed as the target looms nearer, but robot sensors also have lower spatial and temporal resolution than the millions of foveal or tactile receptors, which increase resolution with high rates of identical spikes due to increased motion near the target (see *Fig. 5.2*).

Computational delays increase with desired increases in grasp accuracy, caused by algorithms that calculate target location, creating feedback latencies that become problematic in close proximity to the target. The situation is different in biological systems, where a division of labor in serial arrays eliminates the central computational data load that

---

[432] Zheng, Y. & Qian, W-H. (2004) Intl. J. Robotics Res. 24:311; Kehoe, B., Berenson, D., Goldberg, K. (2012) 8th IEEE Intl. Conf. Autom. Science Engin. p. 1106.

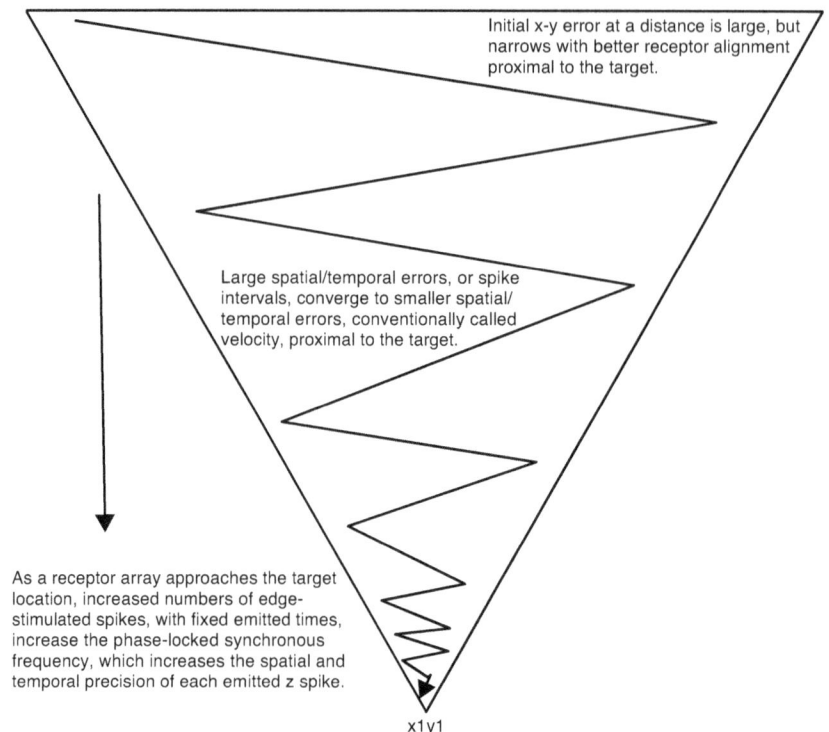

Fig. 5.2: A fine spatial grain of sensory surface receptors focuses, by increasing spike rate in specific receptors and thus spatial and temporal resolution, as the target nears.

could accrue with high spike rates or frequencies, because serial reduction of spike rates occurs in convergent circuits, in which identical z spikes synchronize proximal-distal spike locations and emitted times to retain proximal resolution (*Fig. 5.3*).

Computed signals also need to be converted from analog to digital form, shaped, multiplexed via any of various methods, held in a buffer temporarily; the signal is then converted into information packets of appropriate length, with an input address, output address and a time stamp to direct it to a processing location, algorithm step or to temporary memory.[433]

---

[433] Merolla et al., Osswald et al., op. cit. Chap. Four.

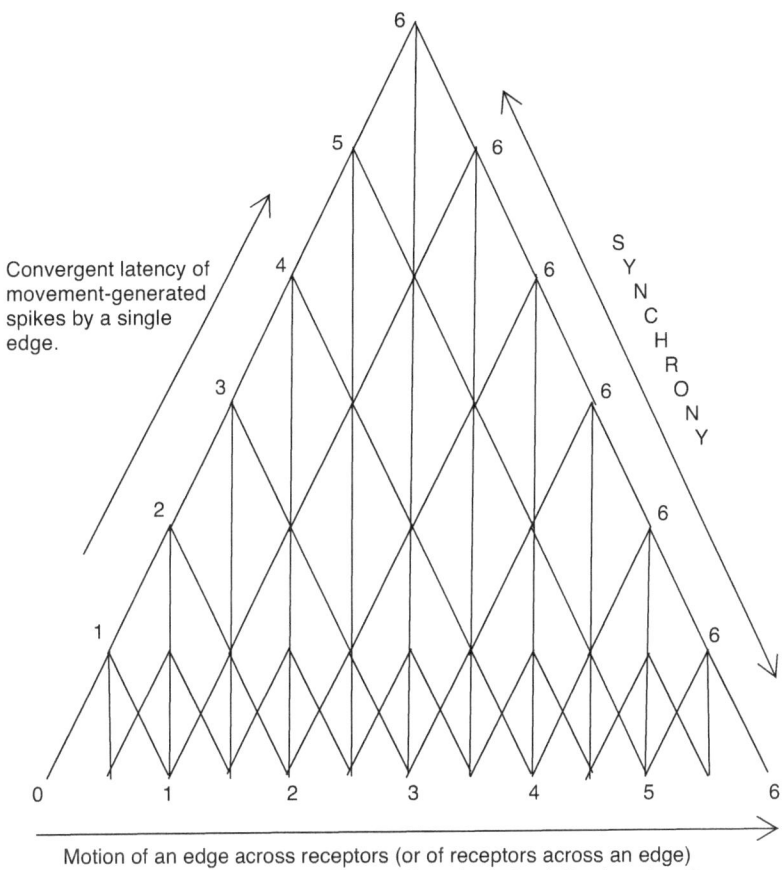

Motion of an edge across receptors (or of receptors across an edge) sequentially synchronizes spikes at aligned proximal-distal x-y locations.

Fig. 5.3: This model summarizes much complex and overlapping circuitry. An initial moving edge at '0', spatially and temporally summates, increasing latency at serially convergent synapses. With sustained edge motion, increased precision is possible, due to the attachment of new edge-stimulated RGC spikes to older spikes that distally converge to synchronize after 80-100 msec duration of edge movement. Conventional temporally coded feedback would require looping delays that last at least the same time, but motion-induced synchrony at distal perceptual cortex and at the proximal receptor has a higher spatial and temporal precision defined by higher spike rates at the stimulated RGC and receptor. This synchrony of delayed perception and receptor precision is essential to explain Fig. 3.1 or batting a baseball; it may also function in V5 cortex and in sensory-motor systems such as the cerebellum.

These computational procedures all introduce delays and programmed complexity that in neurons, would impede the stepwise coordination of spike emitted times (these micro-memories are like stored bits in computer chips), which temporally and spatially synchronize at synapses in repeated 2D arrays. The identical spikes here have no information or destination code, but use labeled neuronal circuits to impedance match types of peripheral information with convergent cortical perceptual areas. Because computer problems are solved by dividing and conquering, processors require a master clock to coordinate activities among hardwired and programmed silos of knowledge. A central processing unit executes software instructions sequentially, taking the place of identical z spikes that traverse 2D arrays, which continuously update sequential latencies at serially convergent synapses at any synchronous instant. Even if asynchronous event timing creates informational packets in lower-bandwidth neuromorphic chips, due to synchronized calibration at higher levels of processing, the delay of executing stored, coded instructions through reiterative loops, and the coding and decoding of sent information, even though emulating some aspects of neural systems, is a process that is still relatively inefficient.

Deep learning uses algorithms to learn new patterns by comparison with a pattern in memory or a programmed goal. This requires software and hardware that emulates neural networks with many modifiable 'synapses' in layers and many iterations of the same convolutional algorithm that stochastically converges on, or learns, the correct solution.[434] Repetition of the algorithm through the layers of the network extracts common features, abstractions or points of distinction in the stimulation data. Coupled with a pooling layer, transformation of this in-

---

[434] LeCun et al., op. cit. Chap. Three.

formation to a 1D temporally coded stream can find sensitive details and be insensitive to large irrelevant variations that may impede perceptual constancies.[435] The repetitive application of the same general purpose learning algorithm, not predefined or precise rules of inference on labeled data, is the most important factor that improves the extraction of image features or abstractions. Only with time and resource intensive computation is human performance approached and now surpassed for complex, repetitious medical diagnostics or recognition of commonalities in highly detailed images; human memory and cognitive abilities are taxed by large amounts of detail. The learning algorithm works eventually because temporally coded binary information that passes through selective simple off-on digital switches is of much lower dimensionality than the weighing factors that adjust selectivity by back-propagation of outcomes from one layer as inputs to the next layer. The repetition of the general purpose algorithm, in effect, adjusts the filtering connections by comparing recurrent results with respect to preset goals programmed into the network. This iterative procedure that eventually learns via feedback reduces to the distributed process here, which depends on the repetitive identity of 1D z spikes to synchronize, at the same time instants, sensory detail with a distally filtered, generalized, abstract z location/time reemitted in an aligned RF (*Fig. 4.6*). The z spikes here vary rate and least-time synchronize proximally-distally within reemitted windows of time, but do not encode a temporal stream of data; rather multidimensional proximal data phase-locks with reemitted distal identical 1D z

---

[435] In fact, visual image stability can be extracted by pooling, or averaging the variable image positions over time; in LeCun et al., op. cit. Chap. Three.

spikes in a continual process. The brain does not use stereotypical algorithms on detailed data that stochastically converge on a solution over time, but rather uses stereotyped anatomy to instantly filter, converge and synchronize 1D z spikes. Recognition in the paradigm here occurs because peripheral information synchronizes most rapidly in an embryonically predefined route through 2D surfaces, refined by later learning with very few reiterations, to any of many specific IT clusters of cells (*Fig. 4.5*).

Because multi-sensory and spatial and temporal convergences occur in temporal cortex, identical least-time distal spikes synchronize object categorization and binocular stereo perception with the sustained edge-stimulated spatial pattern of spikes generated by the specific stimulus object. Due to the proximal-distal time synchronized by sustained sensory spikes at any instant of time, multiplexing and decoding of binary-coded edge information is not required distally. But the intrinsic properties of repetitive time embodied by identical z spikes at a gamma frequency, also spatially stabilize the 1D convergent perception of proximal 2D information. Because proximal-distal synchronization requires serial spatial and temporal summation, the enduring perception of proximally defined precision and distally perceived spatial stability is due to the contextual change of moving spikes from sustained fixed x-y edge-emitted times, to continuously displaced z locations that converge latent z times without any coded x-y information.[436] Anatomical convergence of the FEM-generated spikes to unshifting cortical

---

[436] As discussed in Chapter Three, the response of a V1 cell to multiple types of stimuli does not indicate multiplexing of information (Li et al., op. cit. Chap. One; Prince et al., op. cit. Chap. Three; Read & Cumming, op. cit. Chap. Three), but an impedance-matched responsiveness to any stimulus.

clusters of cells (Chapter Three) does not create the perception of spatial stability; in fact a several hundred-fold cumulative neural divergence to many feature-responsive IT cells occurs. But sustained high RGC spike rates distally reduce nominally separate object recognition, edge-detection, binocular stereovision and image stability processes to a convergence of identical z spikes in multiple synchronized 1D z spike streams of moving locations/time.

The impedance match of internal brain perception with external reality, here requires synchronization in serially repeated modules of synaptic logic, which correlate the plastic facilitation of spike reemission with any external logic, whether imposed by social hierarchies, various religious mysticisms, abstruse mathematics or the specific steps learned to plant and harvest particular types of food. Increments of logical change easily adapt in human evolution despite the inconsistencies of archaic logic when contrasted with a current logical perspective. The current perspective is always the most meaningful even though this was true at every incremental step leading up to the modern view. So how does the brain cope with different logics without mixing them in distal convergent perceptual time? 1) Instead of averaging many spikes over time to standardize measurements for repeatability, the aligned, connected emitted and latent z spike locations/times are perceived within each synchronous increment in time; 2) Conscious cognition uses stereotypes to quickly organize evolving external reality into established hierarchies; 3) Labeled receptors select for the convergence of identical spikes within labeled RFs that synchronize sustained, high rates of sensory information with delayed perceptual time at any synchronous instant of proximal-distal time.

One can test for differences between the theory and hypotheses here and conventional information transfer. In a synchronous, impedance-matched neural system, if *Figs. 4.2* and *5.3* hold, reemitted spike rates do not depend on the quantity of information encoded by bit rate or bandwidth. Rather spike frequency in perceptual cortex depends on the distance between specific synapses in serial temporal and spatial summations, also known as the resonance frequency of the enclosed distance, area or volume.[437] That perceptual intensity increases with greater volumes of spikes on synapses that remit faster, also confounds with greater temporal resolution, is not temporal coding, but consistent with fixed spike times that quickly reemit and summate at greater numbers of synapses, so synchronizing nearby populations of neurons. Here, 1D z spikes with no multiplexed 2D information, converge and diverge at synapses in serial 2D surfaces; spike frequencies temporally synchronize locations (*Fig. 4.2*), rather than transmitting temporally coded, stable information (perhaps requiring error correction) that distally reconstructs a sensory image. The expanded size of distal RFs and the increased quantities of synapses and cells in the RFs, maintains frequencies inversely proportional to RF area and the neural z distance and concomitant z spike latency to that RF. This lower maintained frequency skips repetitive sustained proximal spikes from the same edge, but endures as the synchronously perceived z dimension. Subliminal peripheral spikes with high spatial and temporal resolution are perceived over any fixation period, if serially aligned in the same RF and in proximal-distal z synchrony (*Fig. 3.3*).

---

[437] Lachaux et al., op. cit. Chap. Three; Varela et al., op. cit. Chap. Four, Lea-Carnall, C., Montemurro, M,, Trujillo-Barreto, N., Parkes, L., El-Deredy, W., (2016) PLoS Comp. Biol. $\underline{12}$:e1004740.

Here, a spike at a terminal synapse in an IT cell cluster is not a sparsely coded or multiplexed version of peripheral stimulus information. An integration of the data of experiments detailed in this and previous chapters leads to the theory that each RF-aligned z spike has intrinsic properties of an initial emitted time, reemitted sequentiality and distal latency, which by continuous movement, synchronize rapidly changing information and high spike rates at the sensory surface, with moving, identical z spike locations that traverse serial 2D surfaces during the sustained fixation period, as shown in *Figs. 4.2-4.6* and *5.3*. That these timing properties are intrinsic, means that they are not permanently assigned or coded or tagged onto the spike, but alter over changing contexts of convergent time and distance, in which anatomical selection by synapses, such as in the AM area of IT cortex that responds to facial features, determine reemitted spike rates. Current experiments require standardized conditions that cannot adequately test contextual time because the presumed information stably stored in temporally coded spikes does not change over time or distance. But experiments have shown that a synchronous context emerges when single sequentially emitted spikes sustain as multiple spikes over distance.[438]

The logic of synchronous time here requires orthogonal serial arrays of both the observed and the observer's retinal surfaces. The dimensional reduction is not of peripheral information, but a convergence of fixed emitted times, of identical 1D spikes continuously synchronizing as moving z distances/ latencies to topographical surfaces, a division of labor at serial layers of convergent synapses that reemit from the synchrony of input spikes. Sustained

---

[438] Traub et al., Brovelli et al., both op. cit. Chap. Four.

instants of real-time receptor precision at high spike rates, as moving z locations and times that endure to become latent distally, adjust synchronized frequencies to distal locations rather than data rates, to repetitively link via moving 1D spikes, serial hardwired RF-aligned proximal-distal synaptic loci.

Because the least-time, rapidly reemitted frequency at any serially convergent synapse is a property of the encompassed axonal distance from a synchronously emitting synapse in an orthogonal surface, at a consistent repeatable spike speed, the emitted time is fixed and defined even at the latent distal location where recorded (*Fig. 4.1*). If the emitted spike time did not stay fixed as it moves to the rapidly synchronizing synapse, its distance/latency (integrating, or confounding, both speed and the constant ratio at serial synaptic locations) also would not be repeatable. The concept that the time unit increases with distance traversed, also requires a static fixed emission time that lasts as it moves to the distal location, as an intrinsic feedback comparison. 1D synchrony is latently perceived due to the continual movement of z spikes through the same x-y locations in proximal-distal arrays, so repeated emitted times phase-lock in a continuous process of moving locations/times that integrate moving times at distal locations in a single dimension of time.

Although standardized time and distance provide a reference for measurement and comparison, standardized time and distance units depend on metaphysical assumptions that govern the validity of the quantitative approaches used. As demonstrated here, if objective data do not quite explain the neural phenomena studied, this indicates that the assumptions used to interpret data should change. The mix of current experimental results does not create understanding of anticipatory spike synchronization, confounding a temporal phase advance that is actually due to a spatial phase shift, measured in a component of an averaged synchronization frequency at an electrode location.[439] Advances in phase timing in a component of an averaged frequency or LFP are not an acausal timing relationship, but are due to a shift from the reference electrode location. For example, measurements of phase reversal recorded in the same time period are linearly related to recording electrode depth at the same 2D cortical location.[440] Standardized time is therefore not sufficiently parsed with respect to 2D recording locations in current analyses. Here, synchronization between locations requires sequential emitted-reemitted lags of identical 1D z spikes, without multiplexed 2D information, but correlated with the same repeated x-y loci in serial arrays.

Should the convention of three spatial and one time dimensions be modified so each spatial dimension has an associated time dimension? Current structural and neurophysiological experiments support a change in metaphysical interpretation so that the unitary time dimension scales with spatial extent. Standardized time used for temporal coding and information theory confuse the analysis with a stabilizing complex of perhaps excessive data.

---

[439] Peruse Scholarpedia illustrations of phase lag for 'Synchronization'.

[440] Matias, F., Gollo, L., Carelli, P., Bressler, S., Capelli, M., Mirasso, C. (2014) Neuroimage 99:411; Brovelli et al., op. cit. Chap. Four.

Science Friction
And the Evolution of Complexity

The social hierarchies that exist in science and elsewhere, give status to those who are deemed to have abilities required for the position. Knowledge is built upon a very rigorous system of logic built up over many years, a house of cards or an indestructible temple, depending on one's point of view. Essentially the same causal logic and empirical reasoning, enabled by the same language, are used in all levels of human hierarchy. Thus natural competitive mechanisms based on evolution, allow those who have motivation to jump through hoops correctly, to supersede peers using the same logic tools.

So what happens when a new item of knowledge is found that does not conform with the structure of previous epistemology? It has to be tested to make sure that it is new knowledge. This role falls to the knowledgeable mavens of science. The new knowledge may be based on a new Scientific Revolution, and to incorporate it into current knowledge it has to be made to conform to the dominant means of expressing that knowledge, although it is based on new data or a reinterpretation of old data. This scientific imperialism is a tried and true process, tested in colonial conquests of what, to European discoverers, was a strange new plant, animal, or technique, but which actually developed due to its cradle in a geographically isolated environment. An example was the discovery of curare, the muscle relaxant used for many centuries by South American Indians as a hunting poison, and extracted by them from its natural source with an amazingly sophisticated process, considering the limited resources of the rainforest. Social imperialism takes discoveries such as curare and reiterates the extractive procedure in a standard form, but is destructive of unique cultures that make the idiosyncratic discoveries that Science is credited with. This process is justified on the grounds that it is better for civilization as a whole, even though aboriginal originality is diminished by the larger and more influential social network it now interacts with.

This same attitude holds true today. Established science is not capable of integrating without reinterpretation data that contradict the paradigms established over many years, and may initially resist new discoveries that challenge traditional beliefs. Orderly science likes a standardized, unchanging rectitude. Logic develops in a highly controlled way, based on previous scientific knowledge, or in a less organized serendipitous process in unexplored areas, where current knowledge is deficient. Any alternative logic, for example acupuncture, is quantified in the form of the dominant scientific paradigms or left mystical. Any interesting ideas, which develop mostly by integrating novel influences at the boundaries of the discipline, are bastardized into current scientific paradigms. Imperialistic attitudes from the middle ages are present in a science in which standardization requires tradition is preserved. Novel discoveries are based on the incremental development of originally simple assumptions and facts, resulting in an increasingly complex amalgam of new data. This is in tune with the exponential information overload created by the increased numbers of workers in the sciences; and the emphasis on computational workability, which thrives on complex detail, or hides complexity with statistical interpretations of big data.[441] The many degrees of freedom of multiple, complex analyses of the same phenomenon cannot predict the future with much confidence, but each analysis is internally logical, if full of probabilistic inferences.[442]

Science has steadily become more bureaucratized in the years since WWII, as it has acquired governmental and other institutional funding. In keeping with bureaucratic principles, methods, procedures and terminology are systematically repetitive. Students are trained in rigidly defined methods and greater amounts and complexities of technology. These limit acceptable logic to the incremental step-by-step additions to present tried and tested techniques, tending to inhibit large innovations that

---

[441] There may be a similarity to hierarchy theory, for example in Salthe, S. (1985) Evolving Hierarchical Systems, but the complexity of conventional hierarchy theory seems too narrowly defined. Here, it encompasses not just biological reductionism, but computational and mechanical complexity resulting from repetitive reductionist scaling.

[442] Stirling, A. (2010) Nature $\underline{468}$:1029; are complexity and probabilistic inferences a necessity when dealing with massive information?

could emerge from different assumptions and outlying approaches. Innovative thinking in science has become the abode of those just educated enough to combine naive with sophisticated knowledge, as maturing students are wont to do, but not so well-trained that patterns of thinking become stereotyped, which is defined as expertise. Patterns of thinking are circumscribed, as one presumes that the logic and the language of one's training are correct due to many years of use, to be used as a stepladder for further scientific advance.

Creative questioning of the logical foundations of one's specialty seems undisciplined and can be labeled as muckraking; it is also outside of the realm of expertise of peers. The scientific hierarchy emulates the historical structure of science, which emanates from the fundamental science established by the few Newtons and Galileos and is perceived to be more enduring than the trial-and-error experimentation of everyday experience. Because many scientists at the top of the hierarchy have little time for creative, hands-on science, they may solicit for new ideas. Professors can exploit the best of these ideas, because they have the funding, influence and status that allows them to get ultimate credit for expanding the idea concretely. The idea may be speculative in unpredictable ways; the amount, type and complexity of information and how it is assembled at the source determines its bent. But rewards for volunteered ideas are better than involuntary acquisitions. Big-time science now requires hype as a competitive edge, and the attraction of the press for heroic achievements by stereotypical scientists at the top of the hierarchy, has more public appeal than the origins of a line of research in an unimportant research associate or student's 'naive' but fresh view. The young Einstein and Newton were able to have unrestricted expression, free of credit-diffusing and censoring hierarchical structures, when they imagined and developed their best ideas.

There is a presumption in science, as there is in our democratic society, that everyone has equal information and that more competition is better, for this is the efficient way to make scientific discoveries. However, because competition requires contestants with uniform training and information, limited originality occurs within the bounds of a discipline. In science as in government and large corporations, standardized procedures and training makes any worker replaceable with any other worker. The quest for consistency in science not only allows new techniques and ideas to spread very quickly, it also allows unethical tactics to evolve, which is a democratic need to even the playing field. In the social structure of modern science, strategies exist for distributing credit with various subtle and blunt forms of plagiarism, to be discussed in more detail.

The 'correct' behavior encouraged by scientific standardization can allow a plethora of unproductive behaviors to exist for long periods. Following directions with tried and tested techniques based on the wrong presumptions and interpretations of data can result in years spent on blind work that result in negative findings, necessitating complex or contradictory restatements of the initial hypothesis. One must not underestimate the role of serendipity in finding original results, but explanations of complex findings require a theoretical simplicity at a less reductive level. To study a problem methodically in minute detail may result in data of little importance, but the prospect that it may be found significant motivates researchers onward. Due to rapid innovation, experimental findings may become out of date, of reduced importance, or a crux for further development as more data accumulates.

Criticism of an overriding paradigm of, for example, information theory in neuroscience, may be labeled as 'anti-science'; but is an objective necessity, due to stereotyped thinking and territorial biases. Because convoluted and complex thinking can make a long trail of logic curve in uncorroborated ways, and due to highly structured disciplines, one may not be able to detect that one has asked the wrong question. While the logic may be sound within local bounds, contributing to a provincial factionalism, attempts at a strategic logic that projects outside of a person's specialized knowledge, may be completely dissociated from the tactical reality that any specialist experiences. This strategic logic may be based on current or new assumptions, interdisciplinary concepts in other areas that have different names, theoretical considerations, design permutations for future experiments, or data aggregated or interpreted in new ways. If one doesn't know that the milk that one consumes comes from a cow (real data), rather than an interposed layer such as the milk container (rocket-science equations), specialization can impede strategic progress.

The presumptions that couch one's research may be questionable, but not within the highly circumscribed limits of one's research specialty. If one discovers a dissonant surprising result, how to challenge the dominant paradigm held by leading scientists in the field? One would likely have to follow up the implications of inconsistent but believable results into other areas, to find whether the alternative interpretation has further implications. While it may be possible that a single experiment overturns prevalent scientific views, more probably the interconnected examination of several experiments that show inconsistency, is necessary to affect the assumptions that ground dominant paradigms. Increasingly complex research, based on loyal adherence to traditional paradigms, should be challenged, but can't unless one has greater evidence for an alternative. For the z section concept originating here, one must not only reinterpret spikes as moving locations that are also fixed instants of time, but provide a better explanation for current and past experiments. A viable theory has to be more than abstractions piled on hypotheses, it has to be parsimonious and logically consistent, and refute the concept that information is temporally coded and transferred to cortex, where it reconstructs the visual image on retinotopic maps as statically perceived by the organism. Information theory explicitly quantifies, but is deficient otherwise.[443] The alternative here uses analyzed components of time to show that spikes synchronize cortical perception with peripheral information. That spikes are fixed times and mobile locations rather than coded data, may reduce the complex interaction of perceptual biology and informational physics.

Information is a measure of complexity in computer science, but also is a measure of entropy, as based in Shannon's theory. Information transmitted by stochastic firing, increases with 'full response entropy', but this same information is degraded by 'noisy entropy'.[444] Information is an oxymoron that increases with variable spike timing, and also in-

---

[443] Simon, F. (2014) Wired Magazine 22(1):27. Quantitation creates excesses that need to be balanced by old-fashioned thinking.

[444] For further explanation see Dayan, P. & Abbot, L. (2001) Theoretical Neuroscience, p. 123 ff., or standard engineering references.

creases with the temporal precision required of input spikes to make a synapse fire onward spikes.[445] The different ways to calculate information render it too debatable to be used as a consistent standard across studies. However here, the complexity in a natural image vastly simplifies if spikes do not code information, but move the retinal location of external, RF-aligned object edges. The habitual use of the term 'sparse code' is a speculation that has not specified a standard; the word is in use even though a coding mechanism and/or 'hash table' have not explained away spike variability. The analysis of spikes as a temporal informational code would complicate here, the simplicity of the multi-functional z spike, when analyzed as fixed times at sequential locations. The use of multiple time components here synchronizes reductive z spike times with the delayed phenomenology of perception (*Fig. 4.2*).

Much effort, time, and money can be expended on minute experimentation, to be sure of repeatability. One must attack a problem with different techniques to make results robust, but uninspired science can result from following protocols. Improvements, such as analyzing the connectivity of single neurons within a context of many neurons, may increase the precision of data over the averaging techniques currently used. But the data has to be aggregated and interpreted with correctly derived assumptions. One could also have ten coauthors for this book; could a consensus or a median view allow original thinking to emerge? Experts espousing varied views and of multiple disciplines tend to talk past one another in territorial layers of sophistry. Integrating fundamentals with multiple disciplinary fields requires

---

[445] Mastronarde; Schnitzer & Meister; Usrey & Reid; Reinagle & Reid; Butts et al.; all op. cit. Chapter 3.

adaptability, creativity and the ability to see commonalities without an increase in inefficiency and complexity. The interdisciplinary regularities found may create a metaknowledge.[446]

Reductionism creates blinders of excessively restrictive formalization, trapping one within a myopic view, hindering the insight to see beyond step-wise incremental logic. A current way to deal with increased reductionist complexity is with simulation and modeling in systems biology, but conclusions may be based on trial-and-error hindsight, or unrepresentative factors may be manipulated, which may also be indirectly sensitive to other changing factors. This complexity can hide a plethora of disparate details with large gaps where knowledge is not yet available, and mistaken complex material can masquerade as legitimate, in concert with the high entropy and 'chaos' of highly complex systems. Modularization and filtering can simplify large amounts of data into more tractable entities. Or continual data inputs may drive transitional correlations; as the data sample increases over time, averaging trends scale up from variable current data; more data requires massive computational power.[447]

Very complicated explanations may not be understood at a single time by one brain;[448] this can result in failures due to vaguely seen interactions. To make complexity understandable, one is compelled to create a theory suggested by correlations in much

---

[446] Evans, J. & Foster, J. (2011) Science 331:721.

[447] Anderson, C. (2008) Wired Magazine 16(7):108. To discover trends, without hypotheses and models that attempt to find causes, is limited to correlational data that require interpretation.

[448] This is similar to the empirical ability to remember a number of only 7 + or -2 digits, in Miller, G.A. (1956) Psychol. Rev. 63:81.

data. But there is an overwhelming tendency to put that which is not understood, to a further abstract and/or complex level; this added layer may provide a better vocabulary to understand the material, but it can also mask with an obscurant facade.[449] Interdisciplinary specialists, making consensus decisions with misaligned logics, can create a systemic increase in complex interactions. It should be obvious that there has been a competitive compulsion by scientists to delve further into anatomical, physiological and biochemical complexity, bypassing future simplifying basics that may better explain the brain's mechanisms. Can microcosmic metaknowledge create a comprehensive theory that is also logically consistent and 'simple'? While discovering ultimate mechanisms that explain large scale phenomena is invigorating and an ultimate aim, most reductionist investigations have explanatory gaps,[450] so compelling further study, resulting in increased quantities of data, a process that creates exponentially more questions ad infinitum, but which temporarily satisfies curiosity, exploratory innovation and the need to alter current reality.

Can interdisciplinary collaboration among subfields, or between disciplines themselves, open up inhibiting influences on creativity and logical consistency? Not if the disciplines in question are so stiff with jargon and set protocols that jamming them together is not a synthetic blend but a translation of one in terms of the other. This occurs in biophysics and

---

[449] Kristof, N. (2014) New York Times, Feb. 16, Sunday Review, p. 11; this critic speaks generally about the tendency for academics to create barriers to entry, by using language that is meaningless gibberish. Increased hierarchical complexity of expression is used to hinder access to a common understanding from lower levels.

[450] Brenner, S. (2010) Philos. Trans. R. Soc. Lond. B Biol. Sci. **365**:207; static snapshots do not create a dynamic model of the cell.

psychophysics; in the latter, measurements of perceptual detectability produce psychometric data that are non-linearly condensed in the Weber-Fechner law.[451] For example, one adds a physical quantity, such as weight onto muscle, in increasing amounts; the increases create neural responses that are just noticeable perceptually. This graduated response to a large stimulus range is perceptually and physiologically stable, in that changes are detected without saturating the limited spike rates of neurons that input higher cortical stages (*Fig. 5*). This impedance match is embodied in the maximal RGC rate of a few hundred spikes/sec, while measurements of stimulus magnitude range over a thousand-fold, as stated in Chapter One.

This stable response linearity that hides within psychophysical non-linear power laws is due to biological limiters, such as pupillary diameter and neuronal adaptation, which reduce sensitivity to change at large luminance magnitudes and increase sensitivity to change at low luminance magnitudes. The power law sensory response is sensed perceptually as additive and linear; spike rate increases magnitude with increased stimulus intensity. However, allowing spike rate to adapt to any stably maintained magnitude, over many orders of stimulus magnitude, results in a lower spike response that is graded and non-saturating. Adapted spike rates are obviously not coding absolute stimulus magnitudes.

A similar adapted spike rate at any stabilized stimulus magnitude may have statistical properties that preserve current information-based paradigms, if

---

[451] See Johnson, K., Hsiao, S., Yoshioka, T. The Neuroscientist (2002) $\underline{8}$:111, for a view of the history of psychophysical law. The non-linearity is due to the effect of multiple factors.

multiple time scales of spike train analysis can be a multiplexed code of subtle changes in sensory context.[452] Measured increases in spike rate integrate the dual analytical quantities of stimulus intensity and rate of change; here, these two properties are not multiplexed as a code, but are dimensionally reduced to identical 1D z spikes, similar to rods and blue-stimulated cones that converge to and affect spike rate emanating from the same bistratified RGC, described in Chapter Three.

Increasing spike rate due to looming intensity is also seen in the electroreceptor responses of electric fish, in which spikes adapt extremely quickly to the distant speed of the stimulus. The same spike response to both distant stimulus speed and size, causes a low spike rate to increase as stimulus distance decreases. When the stimulus is nearer, the sustained rate increases in response to the rapid change in stimulus location, or increased speed.[453] Here, we ascribe this increase as necessary for rapid serial summation of spikes to perceptual stages of cortex, which coincides with a more acute perception of an increased spike rate that has a higher emitted-time resolution. Perception of stimulus speed is sensed as a more rapid succession of spike emitted times, at several hundred spikes/sec, a rate due to the shifting locations and increased numbers of electroreceptors stimulated nearer the stimulus. This is similar to looming optic flow in vision, which

---

[452] Baccus & Meister, op. cit. Chap. One, and in Neuron (2004) $\underline{42}$:5, discuss these issues; Fairhall, A., Lewen, G., Bialek, W., deRuyter van Steveninck, R. (2001) Nature $\underline{412}$:787; and Brenner, N., Bialek, W., deRuyter van Steveninck, R. (2000) Neuron $\underline{26}$:695 discuss informational issues that result from adaptive rescaling, in which similar output to any stimulus magnitude must sparsely code magnitude.

[453] Clarke, C., Naud, R., Longtin, A., Maler L. (2013) PNAS (USA) $\underline{110}$:13624.

causes spike rates to increase. At longer axonal distances, slow adapted spike rates are not only metabolically efficient over time but the synapses converge spikes into reduced rates of 1D z perceptual stability. This reduced spike frequency is similar to the redshift to longer wavelengths as the universe expands, which, as argued earlier, cannot be called a locally sensed instant of speed, but is a longer, spatially stable distance/time ratio. The constant c scales proximal-distal distance/time and perception.

Anatomical division of labor between small receptor RFs and large perceptual RFs, enables orders of magnitude changes in intensity to be sensed peripherally, which are not transmitted centrally to a decoder. As Laughlin (1989, op.cit. Chapter Four) writes, the nonlinear reduction in spike rates allows most changes in stimulus intensity to be in the middle of the linear response range. Less common changes in intensity are at either end of that range, so that any stimulus change elicits new spikes. These peripherally generated spikes x-y align with lower rates of perceptual spikes, via convergent emitted times that synchronize in the same z section over neural distance, as in *Figs. 4.2 and 5.3.*

A seeming nonlinearity also is shown in luminance measured in space, which is an order of magnitude more intense than the 100-fold range reflected back from 2-dimensional representations of that space in artwork or photos. The surface pigments on paintings and photos reduce reflected intensities by orders of magnitude (unlike a mirror), to show subtlety in the picture's shading due to lack of sensory saturation. These reflective properties are selected by the artist-observer to match the common perceptual invariances of peers. Here, the impedance match of sustained sensory rates and low cortical rates, detects and perceives the range of stimulus intensities without coding them,[454] by simply synchronizing z spikes over neural distance (*Fig. 4.2*).

Different psychobiological techniques[455] that measure the same phenomenon, may also have dissimilar results.[456] Combining techniques (and vocabularies) may handwave over discrepancies. But the brain impedance matches peripheral response to both stimulus intensity and its rate of change as a single combined perceptual dimension, as stated for 1D z spikes, without multiplexing. In contrast, iterative scientific analyses alter vocabularies, which causes increased complexity layered on simpler previous levels of innovation, to maintain cognitive stability.

The use of consensus or standardization in science, also does not respond well to an eccentric intuition that tries to push a new concept into consciousness; the vague idea may require altering or inventing inflexibly defined words, for communicability.[457] The logic of words and equations that we have associ-

---

[454] 3-dimensional to 2-dimensional nonlinear compressions reduce measured light intensity ratios from 1000:1 to 100:1 from a surface, so that subtle contrasts become visible by, for example, shortening the exposure time of a photo emulsion; or as stated in Chap. One for repeated retinotopic surfaces, limiting light intensity by the pupillary response and reducing z spike rates with neural feedback mechanisms. See Graham, D. & Field, D. (2007) Spatial Vision $\underline{21}$:149.

[455] Single neuron responses vs. measured behavioral characteristics vs. forced choice percepts, as used for smooth pursuit in Chap. Five.

[456] An example are the parallel efforts to sequence the human genome, published in 2001, led by Craig Venter and Francis Collins (Science $\underline{291}$:1304, and Nature $\underline{409}$:860). They used different techniques, resulting in a discrepancy of several thousand genes. Both results were reproducible, but defined by the specific standard used.

[457] For a cogent discussion of the difficulty involved to create a newly-phrased abstraction in quantum theory, such as 'entanglement', see Wilczek, F. (2001) Nature $\underline{110}$:149.

ated into causal chains do not make total sense of the world, so that incremental experiments[458] fill scientific gaps with increased conditional complexity. Reduction seeks simplification; reducing dimensionality is well-known to make complex data analyzable. Rather than using the PCA method to reduce variable and presumptively multiplexed overlapping data, the theory here shows that moving identical z spikes in x-y aligned neurons integrate 2D arrays, by synchronizing emission rate, spike speed and latency between synaptic locations, which synchronize sensory multidimensionality with cortical 1D z perceptions. While masses of data assessed at the same time are prone to spurious correlations,[459] z spikes with no information synchronize as one dimension limited to the same proximal-distal 2D location, in which division of labor between proximal x-y information at a specific time and place correlates with the sequential time of cortical 1D z perception without averaging over time (*Figs. 4.2, 4.4*).

Over time, the numbers of investigators necessary to detail the complex and dynamic ways neurons in the brain are wired has increased; in molecular biology, similar intense efforts have succeeded in sequencing the DNA of advanced mammals. Like miners delving deeper and deeper into the rock to extract smaller and smaller quantities of gold, the increased cost is countered by higher prices caused by unslaked demand. In science, this tendency to expend greater human and economic capital results from, and motivates the development of improved computation and electro-mechanical tools. In the

---

[458] Bussey, J. (2012) Wall Street Journal, Oct. 5, p. B1; discusses the incremental approach in product innovation.

[459] See Wikipedia discussions of 'spurious relationship' and 'correlation does not imply causation'.

primate retina, RGCs are easily categorized into 4 basic types, P and M and Off and On, but beyond these differences, up to 20 types of RGCs are currently distinguishable.[460] Is increased detail necessary to understand the RGC, or does increased informational complexity make the brain less understandable?[461] The diagram below illustrates the complexity that accrues as populations increase, which increase social and economic costs over time, as layers of knowledge build on the previous.

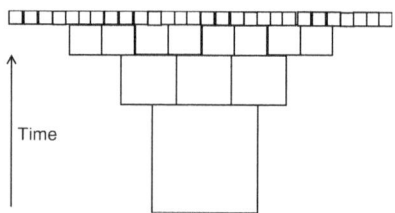

Fig. 6.1: As a technically evolving social group matures, there is a tendency for efforts to sustain that society to become more complex, detailed and intensive. As population increases, the importance of any single member becomes a smaller fraction in the overall complex scheme.[462] In science, paradigms invented long ago are implemented in ever more reductionist detail. At some point the effort, and the payoff from the effort, may balance, so that an asymptote is reached beyond which the degree of advance, balances with much greater costs. Although reductionist ideas, such as the periodic table or the basic neuron, are simple in concept, to explore chemical elements, or neuron types that interact iteratively over time and space, becomes extremely complicated.

---

[460] Field et al. (2007), Masland, op. cit. Chap. Three; the number of different RGC types is similar to the number of cortical visual areas (Wandell et al. op. cit. Chap. One).

[461] Johnson, G. (2014) New York Times, Feb. 18, Science Times, p. D3; discusses the greater difficulty now to make minimal discoveries.

[462] This figure is in concordance with the analysis of several civilizations by J. Tainter, in <u>The Collapse of Complex Societies</u> (1998), in which layers of bureaucracy are added to solve social issues with diminishing effect; resulting in a collapse of the inefficient complex society to a simpler society. Is our society, or scientific methodology, subject to the same inefficiencies that increase with complexity?

A vocabulary created from ordinary experience, when applied to a more exacting scientific analysis, has holes and inconsistencies; with reductionist exploration,[463] an added layer with a more specific terminology is constructed that explains apparent discrepancies; however this interposed layer integrates with more complexity even though simple in its own terms. This is analogous to overlaying two 2D screens with a simple repeated pattern, which creates a more complex Moire' pattern from the layers' interference; or the increase in complexity that can result by repeating a simple algorithm. In particle physics, in contrast to the transparency of massless photons that do not interact electromagnetically, the impacts of heavy particles like mesons and neutrons in accelerators and colliders are used to determine via complex interactions, the reductionist structure of matter. The reductive complexity due to scaling can be managed with principles such as the self-similarity of fractals that scale consistently into the microcosm. Complex neuronal interactions can be lessened with global rules that override local neuronal rules; it is known that groups of neurons control the behavior of individual neurons.[464] Our brain perceives that basic neurons interact in an ex-

---

[463] Examples of reductionist complexity: Of the 500 extremely similar protein kinases in the human proteome, finding the substrate that inhibits one kinase selectively is a problem (from hhmi.org, Jack Taunton data). Also, the multi-step Krebs or TCA cycle, which is the long-known ATP producer in mitochondria, is simple compared to the many regulatory elements, branches and shunts that have been discovered over the years that make a modern metabolic chart much more complicated. Similarly, the many genetic variants that have been found with new techniques to interact complexly in polygenic diseases, such as Alzheimer's, type 2 diabetes, and macular degeneration, have each been found to have little heritable effect, perhaps due to other currently unknown genes and pathways; from Goldstein, D. & Hirschhorn, J.; (2009) New Engl. J. Med. $\underline{360}$:1696, 1699.

[464] Goldman et al., op. cit. Chap. One.

tremely complex system when the presumptions of a single time standard and sequential information, are imposed reductively. In comparison, in the microenvironment of a neuron described in this book, location and time are defined by the synchronized synaptic convergences of identical 1D z spikes, not by aggregating complex coded information.

If layers of rules governing basic underlying monads, e.g. neurons, interact in complex fashion, then this reductive convolution is seen at the perceptual level of organization. That reductive, repeated monads are simple and numerous, shows that logical consistency can result if monads scale without emergent incompatibilities, perceived and analyzed as complexity, that accrue with layering.[465] One may conclude that the intrinsic measures of emitted time, sequential location and synchrony embodied by z spikes, or the spike responses of a single PC in the CB, are actually dimensionally reduced to identical 1D z spikes at RF-aligned 2D surfaces. Matching of impedances is fundamentally necessary for the brain's complex exogenous interactivity.[466] The multiple components of time in *Fig. 4.2* indicate that z spikes, synchronous over z equivalent distances between 2D surfaces, are a contextually flexible dimension. Peripheral informa-

---

[465] Mandelbrot, B. (1977) <u>The Fractal Geometry of Nature</u>. Scaling of self-similar entities can increase complexity into reductive infinity, shown by fractal equations with exponents between 2 and 3 dimensions.

[466] Braun, D., Aertsen, A., Wolpert, D., Mehring, C. (2009) Curr. Biol. <u>19</u>:352; this example of dimensional reduction describes randomly varying learning tasks with many parameters that can be reduced to 1D structures. As discussed herein, neuronal 1D and 2D structural anatomy exists prior to emergent 3D spatial interactions. Because lower dimensional anatomical structures preexist, the "evolved" observer may find novelty in extracting structural invariants from the observer's own increasingly complex reality.

tion is usable without multiplexed, or temporally encoded, strategies to move that information to a central location.

The sequential advance of incremental knowledge deems that Newton's Gravitational Theory was necessary for Einstein to develop his Theory of General Relativity, which explains gravitational mechanics more accurately. As diagrammed in *Fig. 6.1*, a basic scientific theory invented by a Newton, is steadily developed and implemented with more and more sophisticated tools and measurements, in a step-by-step fashion by more and more scientists. In neurophysiology, no epistemological scaffolding has resulted in a consistent theory, though paradigms have periodically popped forth from other scientific and engineering specialties, attempting to make sense of the brain's logic.

The complexity of neuronal interactions is compounded by complex quantitative techniques borrowed from other fields, creating obscuring layers between our perception and the actual phenomena, resulting in complex interpretations of data (this is not true of PCA methods, which support the simple 1D z concept described in this book). The reliance on information theory over decades, has not shown how image information is encoded by spikes, as electrons and photons have done in telecommunications. Neuronal encryption keys have never been found, yet tremendous resources are spent hypothesizing about statistical codes, sparse codes, EEG phase relationships, or spike latency patterns at convergent synapses, which hypothetically must encode information, without proving how these abstract theoretical standards work in neurons. Why? Because information theory is the only formally defined quantitative recipe to code and transfer data.

What seem to be similarities in physical and biological phenomena are oftentimes different in mechanism and in origin.[467] This author protests that intellectual open-mindedness requires more than the dogma of information theory.[468] Other potential interpretations of the brain's mechanisms are not explored due to this dedication to off-the-shelf quantitative methods, whose application to neurophysiology results in usable data, but with the presumption that neurons must use the same logic with which they are analyzed. Standard techniques of quantification can give one a premature but false sense of understanding, thus be tactically acceptable to those seeking a higher publication count, but this scientific 'rigor' creates an intellectual rigor mortis in which more creative and less conventional explanations are not allowed publication by peers guarding an official forum. The dictum garbage in, garbage out holds; if assumptions are not correct, the applied math is a glossy cover up, like a veneer, that gives the impression of scientific rectitude.

Macroscopic data on systems of neurons can separate signal from noise but can only provide average, indirect clues to any single neuron's perhaps counterintuitive logic. Neurophysiological methods select data, nullifying a single spike's precision by pooling with statistics, also by counting spikes in defined time bins at an electrode's location; or by choosing the largest spikes, confounding nearby signals with more distant spikes, or creating conditions that elicit

---

[467] Vogel, S. (2000) J. Biosci. 25:191; discusses examples of biological solutions and analogous human-engineered solutions to the same problem that have qualitative differences.

[468] Compare the opinion piece about scientific dogma and its role in interpreting the data of Alzheimer's disease, by Perry, G., Raina, A., Cohen, M., Smith, M. (2004) The Scientist 18:6.

the most emphatic numbers of spikes, etc. These bias the analysis because the data are preselected, which may cause circular reasoning.[469] This author argues against stepwise increases in complexity within standardized methodologies that preserve aged assumptions; one must favor simple definitions coupled with basic data, in which evidence guides intuition, to detect the brain's overlooked fundamental mechanisms.

The inverted pyramid in *Fig. 6.1* is based on initial simple rules and presumptions devised by past individuals such as Hippocrates, Euclid and Galileo, at initial positions in modern history. Over time, new data superseded old information. New interpretations of old data emerged, such as the Copernican Revolution, in which cosmological analysis showed that the planets did not revolve around the earth but around the sun. The generic success of cumulative knowledge caused better living conditions and increases in human population. This required new measures of competence to create academic hierarchies, in which followers used logical templates to expand knowledge. But by using the same template repeatedly, there is an evolutionary tendency for incremental details to add of declining importance. Data is now so massive and complex that to analyze it awaits the use of large computer resources. This accumulation of changing facts can increase due to more detailed questions, asking the wrong questions and asking the same question from slightly different viewpoints that result in different solutions.

Mathematical techniques exist for finding regularities in massive data, however their success depends on

---

[469] Circular reasoning is discussed in Kriegeskorte, N., Simmons, W.K., Bellgowan, P., Baker, C. (2009) Nature Neurosci. $\underline{12}$:535.

the initial questions that parse the data in useful ways.[470] Historically in physics, it was necessary for Faraday to show that electricity and magnetism interact via fields rather than the action-at-a-distance equations current at the time; Maxwell used Faraday's intuition about fields, based on data, to create symmetrical equations that have been extremely useful over time.[471] Data may also have heterogeneous conditions that invalidate the results.[472] This is especially so in biology, which has large variation and deviation in the data that can mask local precisions. A different explanation like that described here, exposes assumptions formalized as standards, such as a precise spike temporal code transmitted to a location is more useful to synchronize spikes at serial synapses. Further analysis of spikes into emitted, latent and synchronized components, as in Chapter Four, may explain how spike variability in neural populations impedance match sensory data.

Is a step-by-step slog the best way to improve science, based on unchanging assumptions? Or does the quest for scientific consistency apply only to current experimental findings but not old results?[473] Increasing quantities of data, built on historical layers of data, may accumulate a complex result that refuses to give a robust, clear-cut solution to the same question. If reductionist knowledge is dependent on complex interactions, manipulating one

---

[470] Carlsson, G. (2009) Bull. Amer. Math. Soc. 46:255.

[471] Wilczek, F. (2015) A Beautiful Question.

[472] Ioannidis, J., Trikalinos, T., Zintzaras, E. (2006) J. Epidem. 59:1023; Potsopoulos, N., Evangelou, E., Ioannidis, J. (2009) Intl. J. Epidem. 38:1740.

[473] Ioannides, J., Tatsioni, A., Karassa, F. (2010) Eur. J. Clin. Invest. 40:767; how does one update outdated experimental results?

highly specialized area can indirectly introduce instability into other areas where causal connectivity is vague, resulting in a chaos.[474]

To explain causally is problematic at the lowest levels of biochemistry due to the increased complexity of molecular interactions that create a nonlinear systems dynamic at these obscured, indirectly sensed levels.[475] Because we sense reductively by using intermediary instruments, one is forced to make assertions about a biochemical interaction that may not apply outside of highly specified conditions. More generally, any shift, or even slight alteration in an experimental condition changes the experimental results and the interpretations one can make about a phenomenon. As already described by Eyal et al. (op. cit. Chapter Four), integrating the dendritic field and its adjoining axonal spike initiation site in the same model radically alters results, showing that impedance matching is required for synchrony. If the phenomenon being studied has consistently robust results in response to many manipulated conditions, it may withstand the test of time. The novelty of new findings is relative to new conditions and new methods: added layers of complex analysis alter the cognitive environment, causing a form of circular reasoning because the new results are predicated on the use of the new methods.

New techniques in old areas, old techniques in new areas, and new techniques in new areas of research

---

[474] Cause-effect biochemistry exists only in experimental isolation, otherwise complex, inconsistent interactions predominate; see Campbell, T. (2007) The Scientist 21:14.

[475] Huang, S. & Ingber, D. (2006-2007) Breast Disease 26:27 discuss the multitude of molecular interactions that leads to the coherent final state of cancer. Reductive complexity can be acausal such that the order in which factors are added does not affect the result.

churn out increased data that may modify old findings. Increased complexity that accompanies reductionist approaches can hinder due to the unwieldy nature of attempts to manipulate microscopic phenomena with microscopic tools. To explore causal relationships reductively increases the connections among data points that have to be attached, a time-consuming and complex, nonintuitive process. The reconstruction of a sensed image from spikes, or holistic physiology from known molecular interactions, is called the inverse problem and is virtually impossible with current reductionist knowledge and techniques.[476] At some point consistent results may accumulate to create a new theory that is predictive, reducing the need for more experimentation. Here the inverse problem is avoided because z spike locations and times do not reconstruct an image.

Many engineering advances historically have been due to conceptual leaps; over the ages, improving technologies have freed laborers for more productive behaviors. In science, in the interest of thoroughness, there is always the possibility that a great discovery lies just over the horizon if one delves into heretofore unexplored geographical areas, or finds a better animal model to explore a disease, or sees a gap in the reductive complexities of biochemistry or neurophysiology that needs to be filled with new data. Alternative logics, if they improve complex inconsistencies and therefore are not simply tacked onto traditional paradigms, should be allowed to simplify procedures, in a robust fashion. Trial-and-error science, the use of improved approaches to give further insights that invalidate previous results,

---

[476] In systems biology, the view has emerged that the cell, rather than molecules, at a mid-level of analytical abstraction, is more suitable for holistic reconstruction, in Brenner, S., op. cit.

displaces results that may actually still be relevant and may increase transitional difficulties of legacy material with the new. Complex parts may work cooperatively, but may be subject to Braess's Paradox, in which an added conduit to improve flow, can degrade performance of the whole network.[477] More thoughtful methodologies, designed adaptively so that change is factored in, analogous to some consumer software, could reduce the hidden disadvantages of complex activities.

One should interpret increasing complexity as a need to periodically organize information overflow with appropriate protocols. The detrimental effect of massive accumulations of complex data, fights with the tendency for expertise in complexity as a signal of educational status. Averaging data reduces the significance or the hidden sensitivity of any single component. This is relevant here for the hypothesis that z spikes at a local synaptic ensemble, use wavelengths (or spatial intervals) among spikes at nearby locations in the ensemble to stimulate associated memories, rather than using phase differentials of an averaged frequency at an electrode location to code memory. One may use systems science to simplify, preferably as data accumulates rather than after it accumulates, by eliminating data according to preset protocols, to make the future a predictable self-fulfilling prophecy. Can logical developments that increase complexity be remodularized, so that outmoded legacy material is eliminated without completely reconstructing structural underpinnings? There may be a time when the algorithms of information compression or dimensional reduction cannot rescue us from the inevitable tendency to fill space with an increased, unintegrated complexity of

---

[477] Braess, D. (1969) Unternehmensforschung 12:258.

data, sometimes known as spam. This atherosclerotic overload of voluminous material may stabilize knowledge by increasing complex webs of now static information that aggregate over time.

As alluded to, complexity may result from a stepwise application of stereotyped thinking patterns on a substrate that has changed due to previous application of the same thinking pattern.[478] Due to this predictability, it is possible to skip steps to create a more stable state of human thought, so that intellectual energies can be devoted to other areas. The apposition of Darwinian innovative evolution, with unchanging scientific standards, are paradoxes that we have habituated to. That innovation is essentially contextual, now combining inputs from formerly separate disciplines, can be used to adjust future trajectories of thinking to reduce complexity.

The innovative, competitive response, to increase the complexity of knowledge despite a steadily increasing social or monetary cost to do so, is akin to the lack of planning that causes traffic jams as more employees are required for new industries in a local area. Only after subdivisions are already built, shopping malls constructed, new company headquarters erected next to those of other firms, greener substitutes for gasoline instituted, and a complex and long bureaucratic process is traversed, is increased traffic flow accommodated by wider freeways. It takes longer for a population to transition to fewer or smaller commuter vehicles. Many other societal indicators show that increasing complexity slows activity, resulting from an incremental-

---

[478] An older version of this idea is in The Structure of Scientific Revolutions, by T. Kuhn (2nd edition, 1970). Time has allowed its robust reemergence and further development into hypercomplexity here.

ism to which we adapt, such as, increasing the numbers of jurors called to the invasive inquisition now required for jury duty, due to increasingly finicky lawyers, or the tendency for legislatures to enact more, increasingly complex, and less understandable laws. Are social organizations growing to a scale that are impeded by the aggregation of formerly minor factors? An unimportant detail can be unrecognized amid a multitude of other details until it stops traffic on the interstate or brings down an airliner. In engineering, it is a truism that failure rate increases with complexity, which increases with the number of components. The brain has complex wiring but also has redundant modular monads and neurons designed to adapt quickly, each with little effect on the total machine. Modern societies have hidden vulnerabilities untested over time because innovation that increases complexity cannot plug unseen gaps that may result when novel specialized components fail, jamming tuned interdependencies.

The increased innovation in social media and business communication requires mutual assurances and 'trust' to perform well, which disruptive hackers take advantage of. There is an interaction between innovative complexity, and periodically emerging disorder, which is only momentarily resolved by corrective feedback from after-the-fact, delayed solutions. The periodic reassessments that adapt to security disruptions with increasingly complex solutions, only temporarily alleviate these disruptions. Stable lasting solutions that cannot be hacked are not apparent *a priori*. However, unconventional use of big data, in a delayed loop, may find generalizable consistencies that require huge resources to be hacked.

While increased data storage and complexity enables personalized medicine and directed advertising, the tolerance of creative eccentricity has transferred to a mass-market society that uses social media to trend with the latest enterprise. A symptom of crowd behavior is the many times more clinical syndromes in the latest edition of the Diagnostic and Statistical Manual of Mental Disorders, compared to the first edition from the 1950's.[479] The difficulty in revising the fifth edition, published in mid-2013, exhibited the increasingly immobile state that competitive hierarchies are evolving into. Medical specialists, in successive attempts to improve on their forebears, have steadily increased the number of formally defined disorders. What was tolerated as social diversity in the past can be made a legally-binding mental disability in what is a political act for inclusion in the manual.[480] Incremental innovation not only increases the number of defined 'disorders' but elevates and magnifies minor details that allow organizational functionaries to scapegoat individuals into discriminated labels. New disorders, in a stepwise cycle of competition, establish reputations and create more data, but are an increase in formal syndromes, despite ambiguous qualification and quantification of abnormality, an improvement?

Diagnostic hair-splitting has created variants of autism, called a spectrum, one being Asperger's syndrome, which is based on the interaction of many genes. The incidence of autism has increased several times in recent decades; interacting genes cannot have increased expression of the autistic spectrum so quickly and recently. The increased autistic spectrum parallels the increase in DSM-V

---

[479] Carey, B. (2008) New York Times Dec. 18, p. A1.

[480] This vote on what constitutes a psychiatric disorder, and other issues, are discussed in Kupfer, D., First, M., Regier, D. (2002), A Research Agenda for DSM-V.

disorders and in RGC types already described: is spectral variation synonymous with increased social complexity? Genetically defined diverse behaviors may create a tendentious objectivity.[481] Debate on this issue has caused a reduction in the numbers of disorders in a recent DSM-V manual.[482] While outlying eccentricity is necessary for diverse and creative viewpoints, in my opinion it is used as a basis for discriminatory hierarchies in nominally democratic societies, which impose bureaucratic 'standards' to incrementally reduce acceptability in their ranks.

Big-brother tendencies emerge when governing larger groups, creating more subtle definitions of personality 'disorder'. Stereotypes of acceptable behavior create motivation for competitive hierarchies to disqualify, imprison or medicate outliers in the increased spectrum of disorder. An increased need for hierarchical differentiation legitimizes newly invented labels, which are not protested by individuals because they are not organized as groups or trained as behavioral scientists. The legal system and large government and business organizations, contribute to this pedantic misuse of science that profiles individuals into labeled classes, with the stated purpose of fitting personalities for particular job duties and to bias juries favorably.

Academic hierarchies are the most flagrant inventors of the barriers that purposefully hinder upward crea-

---

[481] While differences in the autism spectrum may be sourced in multifactorial genetic interactions (see Vernes, S., Newbury, D., Abrahams, B., Winchester, L., Nicod, J., Groszer, M., Alarcon, M., Oliver, P., Davies, K., Geschwind, D., Monaco, A., Fisher, S. (2008) New Eng. J. Med. 359:22), should the increase in complex variation that is discriminable in larger populations be a basis for modifying definitions of normal standards of behavior?

[482] Carey, B. (2012) New York Times, May 9, p. A11.

tivity. For example, a professor may espouse social media to obtain new ideas that may be useful for new experiments. Yet the researcher's raw data, perused online, has detailed restrictions on its use. A person who can analyze the data with better methodology, has to ask for permission to use the data or face 'plagiarism' charges even with proper credit given. Proprietary entitlement allows principal investigators who do not understand their data to publish outdated interpretations over a long period.

Scientific progress goes periodically bankrupt, stifled by incrementalism, predictable outcomes and standardized interpretations of data. A short-cut solution to the social impediments that retard the invention of creative theories is simply to use group power to acquire innovative theories or attractive ideas outright from individuals. Synergism of ideas, verifiable predictions and logical consistency distinguish a scientific theory from an everyday idea. Yet the hierarchical academic will refer to a well-developed theory as an idea, if submitted by one of lower rank, to justify the acquisition of the theory so that they can develop a more complex or 'correct' version of it. Because a novel idea exists, a scientist may single-mindedly fixate upon it to the exclusion of alternative but less attractive older ideas that would otherwise be just as plausible if more pluralistic goals were important. Ideas are basic to develop experiments and being fluid, can be worded in various ways; so if explicitly defined in the static wording of a copyright or patent, are easily leapfrogged by innovative exploiters. Because scientific standardization deems that exact wording describes a new phenomenon, plagiarism can be glaringly obvious; in fields where description is flexible, such as literature and art, many ways exist to express a common sentiment without stepping on the originators' toes. The peer review process allows authoritative scientists to review articles submitted for publication anonymously; they can apply reworded concepts in any way they want, with no violation of copyright or patent law, and without violating any regulatory authority.[483] I have found that my confidentially submitted intellectual property to a journal had a hidden 'fair-play' use,[484] in that ideas were serially excised as inspiration for others' publications.

Make no mistake, plagiarism, or not being given public credit for a significant idea even though the source is known to the offender, is a tactic with effects similar to sexual harassment, affecting the plagiarized person's subsequent willingness to interact scientifically. This is one reason why plagiarists may pass ideas to others to hide the chain of communication near the originator, as if the idea evolved in parallel. Criticism and other manipulations are used to reduce the significance of the thinker's work, so that s/he is an assistant in a bureaucracy that exploits creative ideas with its superior resources, but in which social conformity is enforced hierarchically. Ethics are secondary because delusional rationalizations, outright but unprovable lies,

---

[483] Lisberger, S. (2013) Cerebrum online 2013:6; states that reviewers are in a position to steal innovative ideas and impede the publications of competitors, but that they should uphold a higher standard. This scientist also thinks that the known scientific fraud and plagiarism is the tip of the iceberg, hidden by those lower in hierarchy from those, such as principal investigators, with the authority to do something about it. I have found that the head of the lab cooperates with senior members who have plagiarized from lower seniority members.

[484] Fair-play allows the use of private intellectual property within limited grounds, such as a columnist including a snippet of copyrighted material in a published criticism of that material. Snipping out single ideas of the many presented in this treatise is not fair unless the author is given credit.

using the color of bureaucratic authority and denial, are required to increase competitive advantage and prevent credit to the hidden source of the idea.

Bureaucratic layers of academic status encourage behaviors like taking elements developed by one of lower rank, adding more complex technical material to give the impression of greater depth, but is really stilted filler that does nothing to advance or increase the value of the achievement, which may have been originally designed to be parsimonious. Discriminatory behavior is used to increase hierarchical importance, by imposing a layer of academic 'code', similar to the use of Latin nomenclature in medicine, which insulates from criticism of plagiarism. Clever glory hogs who steal credit from underdogs displace creative science and should not be in responsible positions for ignoring standards of ethical behavior. While medical doctors take an oath of ethical integrity, no such oath is overtly enforced in academia. In my experience, the enforcement of standards concerning plagiarism by those striving for academic ranking, is rudimentary and discouraged by purposeful delays and the wiles of midlevel lawyers and administrators, who make decisions based on academic biases, despite the official public message that misappropriation of ideas is an ethical offense.

Over-the-line competition uses plagiarism to escape the blinders of traditional science.[485] Recidivist denials and coverups result as those with superior status and ambition take intellectual property from individuals without giving credit. This social imperialism is not restrained by publicized rules, because scientists are presumed to be rational humans, not

___
[485] Charlton, B. (2009) Medical Hypoth. 73:644; one of several commentaries by this author on the epidemic of dishonesty in science.

greedy animals. Academic rectitude hides a knee-jerk resistance to strangers with creative attitude, evidenced as a Jekyll and Hyde rejection coupled with the cheerful theft of diverse ideas permitted by the acquiescence of silence, enforced absence or subservient status. 'Fake it until you make it' may mean acquiring ideas without acknowledgment (a cursory nod?) until already published by the plagiarist. The hope of future advancement is held over students' heads to coerce innovative ideas.[486] This selection on any basis rather than quality,[487] reduces the competition for post-doctoral and higher academic positions, in which alternative views are restrained by consensus thinking, bureaucratic correctness and whether a methodological opponent will be judging one's grant application or reviewing one's publication.

Agricultural monocultures with little plant diversity are bemoaned because they allow incipient diseases to flourish quickly, but the monoculture of traditional science also chokes off individual diversity.[488] This intolerance encourages oversimplifying labels, which are of the same mindset as artificial intelligence algorithms that make inductive conclusions (such as facial recognition) from big data, but with biases that cannot be eliminated.[489] A creative new idea may require partnership with a stereotypical

---

[486] See the article on Alia Sabur, Financial Times (2010) October 2/3, L&A, p. 22. Though this report lacks some details, it reveals academic authority impedes science strategically, by shifting credit tactically from the originator, whose advanced degree is then withheld.

[487] Yariz, N., Ioannidis, J., Al-Ubaydi, D. (2008) PLoS Med. $\underline{5}$:e201.

[488] See Physics Today (2006) $\underline{59}$:13; published are multiple views to the lack of creativity in science, especially W.W. Carter's letter.

[489] Haussler, D. (1988) Artif. Intell. $\underline{36}$:177.

standard-bearer of science, otherwise the heretical 'rebel' is excluded from the academic circle,[490] so that an established paragon can publicize or implement the reworded idea. The creator may get jobs that quickly terminate once useful ideas are extracted. Academics have long used devious means to take over confidential intellectual property.[491]

In a quest for transparency and to confront the issue head on, this polemic argues that plagiarism is partly due to reproducible science and rote learning.[492] Why? Because experiments cannot be repeated unless one can regurgitate instructions and standardized procedures. Standardized training allows anyone to parrot a logically presented idea. Advanced scientific education selects for good learners with good memories, not those with disruptive creativity. Standardized protocols are important for teaching science and are necessary for logical communicability, especially in large collaborations, which allow science to enlarge in scale. If there was a standardized procedure for inventiveness and creativity, as with the artificial intelligence program Verifier,[493] it would be taught, but artificial originality is limited to its programmed inputs. Algorithms can only simulate creativity. This book necessarily limits

---

[490] Kristof, op. cit.

[491] That Graham Bell plagiarized essential information for the invention of the telephone from Elisha Gray's patent application, is another example of theft by academic status. See <u>The Telephone Gambit</u>, by Seth Shulman (2008). Status entitles the theft of original material due to secrecy, cover-ups, and the victim's feeling of intimidation.

[492] Stenflo, L. Nature (2004) <u>427</u>:777; Abbott, A. Nature (2007) <u>448</u>:632; Nature (2010) <u>466</u>:436,438; Chaddah, P. (2014) Nature <u>511</u>:127; these are a continuing series of commentaries in the magazine Nature, on plagiarism and a lack of integrity in much of science.

[493] Rugg, G. & Hyde, J.; this program, described online, uses the scientific method to study the psychological process of doing science.

the amount of data used to derive and support conclusions, while deep learning algorithms are able to digest much more data of greater complexity, using standard assumptions and trainable regimens of logic that validate due to repetition. They can only probabilistically assess the validity of unusual or random data and do not create 'original' insights.

For this author, the convention that neural spikes code information has been a mental block for a long period of time. Because many incremental experiments are based on the assumption that APs transfer information, the inertia of this standard has impeded new ideas such as the theory developed here. Convention may deem that a new theory does not apply because it is not in agreement with vested research or developed by a reputable academic.

Scientists who do not acknowledge misappropriated innovative ideas may categorize the hidden originators into populous slots based on social biases. Assertive plagiarists are allowed to ascend the academic ladder with the covert approval of their colleagues, because the academic machine depends on new ideas and inspiration, from whatever source, for innovative experiments. Science likes to think that it has an amoral, objective motivation without sentiment or overt bias. Courtesy of the well-known book, The Double Helix by James Watson, the result is of vastly greater importance than the secretive and manipulative behavior necessary to achieve it. While scientific methodology can be highly regulated, scientific behavior is not; the pole should point oppositely so that plagiarism does not reduce the motivation for or delay innovations of substance.

A young academic may find that plagiarism is necessary to make an instant reputation; good ideas from an unknown, uncredited source are needed because creativity is not easier with higher rank. To intellectually bushwhack with new trains of thought is tough, but artfully combining design ideas with traditional engineering and science can create new science.[494] Workability demands that novelty be simple, communicable, and achievable with short term effort. However, ideas and insights such as those in the previous chapters require unavoidable periods of months and years to emerge. Small interdisciplinary groups are a way to improve products,[495] making the inception of the creative idea incrementally ambiguous. This is an improvement over traditional hierarchies that use hero-worshiping underlings as an unpublicized creative resource.[496] But major conceptual modifications still require a person's independent questions and assertiveness.

How else is plagiarism legitimized? Formal expression of a concept in technical language is more acceptable than less precise forms, and it is the expressed form of the idea, not the formative idea itself, that is protected by copyright. This presumably allows for its unhindered modification. It also allows assertive exploiters with bureaucratized status to hype correctly 'coded', or rephrased, versions of less formal but influential ideas from hidden sources, thereby usurping credit for scientific or commercial innovations from persons they do not consider to be in their peer group or disciplinary silo, regard as disruptors or competitors, or simply wish to ignore.

___

[494] Schneiderman, B. (2016) The ABCs of Research: Achieving Breakthroughs through Collaborations; this author also espouses simplification as a way to achieve elegant solutions.

[495] Rae-Dupree, J. (2008) New York Times, Dec. 7, Business Section, p.3.

[496] Posner, R. (2007) The Tiny Book of Plagiarism.

Hopefully, while discrete ideas in this book may be criticized, they will not be belittled only to be superseded by more complex versions. One can easily find a minor technicality that improves another's major advance, and so take credit for the whole thing.[497] Because loopholes make it expensive to protect intellectual property, the disfunctional use of inside information to steal credit, or 'scoop', the findings of a more creative person with less financial support, is becoming more prevalent.

Where quantity of publications is important, motivations to maximize grant funding or academic status are more important than thinking through ideas to their end.[498] The emphasis in current reductionist science for incremental, tactical advances, also make tenuous, fragmentary ideations publishable in obscure and even mainstream journals; but to integrate and develop creative ideas in a robust manner requires strategic, substantial leaps of thought.[499]

Along with disguised and obvious plagiarism, other anti-competitive practices such as purposeful misinterpretation, false information and diversionary argumentation have been long present as barriers to entry, which allows opportunists to acquire novel intellectual property from hidden sources. Isn't this public maintenance of a rational image based on the hidden abuse of the plagiarized, primitive and irra-

---

[497] Raymond Damadian patented magnetic resonance imaging, but the person who later improved this imaging without crediting Damadian, won the Nobel prize; in New York Times (2004) March 23 issue.

[498] Ioannidis, J. (2011) Nature 477:529.

[499] Much of Andy Warhol's art, especially his silk-screens of soup cans or of Elizabeth Taylor, illustrates that a standardized product can be altered slightly, many times, a satire on the modern tendency to mass-produce originals, as originals.

tional? The medieval class structure that reinforces the conflation of assertive elitism and hierarchical bias against lower ranks is accepted because stereotypes are used to gauge academic validity. A paper submitted in March 1986 to The Journal of Theoretical Biology, basic to this book, in my humble opinion benefited a few who found an opportunity to reject its publication, only to rapidly rethink the ideas into more 'refined' cybernetic terms. Rewording an integrated idea apparently did not require citing it as a reference, especially since it remained unpublished; this tactic of disassembly and rephrasing may be easy to disguise because scientific experimentation is so fragmentary. In my opinion, persons shielded by prestigious institutions and advanced degrees, with the fuel of anonymous assertiveness, stole credit with hyped phrases and superior attitude, using public funds, at the expense of the unknown person who tried to publish the theory. One submitted idea was used in a patent in a related field.[500] In my opinion, unpublished ideas were also communicated to members of a Psychology Department. It is possible to trace the origin of ideas forensically, especially if the misappropriated ideas are not improved in any creative fashion, but simply passed on to others. This rote approach enables the idea to be preserved over time, its source concealed and credited to more preferable associates, in an environment in which group assertiveness has more legitimacy than the privacy sought by the originator to prevent more plagiarism. Use of peer review to acquire ideas requires that the definition of misconduct expand to include purposeful omissions of credit to advancers of science who are of low visibility.[501] By

---

[500] Embodiments of ideas described here have patent-pending status.

[501] Fanelli, D. (2013) Nature 494:149.

preventing a paper's publication, reviewers can anonymously circulate intellectual property, so that others rather than the originator seem to be the source. Rewording others' ideas is present in other professions but should not be in objective science.

The unpublished 1986 paper used the fixational movements of the eye to sustain RGC spikes. My theory went on to say that successive spatial summation of this fixationally shifting spike input at hierarchical convergent synapses, became a temporal code of spatially shifting information, so that the complete conversion to a temporal code of reduced spike rates created spatial and temporal image stability in large cortical RFs. Larger saccades resulted in perceived spatial stability of the whole visual field in the largest convergent RFs of IT cortex. The evidence for this was based in large part, on successively reduced spike rates at sequential levels of the visual system detailed in Van de Grind et al. (op. cit. Chap. One). This synthesis of ideas to explain spatial stability was original at the time. This book improves that paper with more evidence without proceeding from any other theory. In my opinion, peer review has been corrupted in this case so that anonymous readers monopolize new thinking that they paraphrase, disperse credit for and perform experiments upon, which enhances their careers at the expense and the exploitation of others.[502] Sophisticated plagiarists use an original theory to design experiments that test it, which may lend support to it but without stating that a hidden theory is the actual source. The young Newton, Einstein and

---

[502] Felten, E. (2010) The Wall Street Journal, Feb 5, p. W11, explicitly details more modern examples of flagrant and purposeful sabotage by peer reviewers, to prevent the publication of original ideas. It becomes habitual to disguise sources of ideas that are published; cover-ups become an intellectual exercise, anonymous fraud the norm.

even Crick and Watson, did not have anonymous reviewers with hierarchical or competitive biases. Peer review should not improve quality by rephrased plagiarism or censoring new ideas.

Some scientists have an ego created by their bureaucratic position which allows them to delude themselves as to the true origin of a key idea, because the causal chain may be informally known initially, but the originators do not have hierarchical status.[503] Unfortunately, this unjustified confidence may combine with the impostor syndrome, a belief by important contributors that they are undeserving of rewards. The irrational adherence to primitive hierarchies needs stereotypes and selective biases. So coverups are normal in academia, standards are maintained by facile denials. As published reports state, maintaining a professional veneer may create despotic effects.[504] The scientific hierarchy is as jealous of its privileges and guards its estimable colleagues as effectively now as in previous decades,[505] by official inquiries that divert and dissemble, reactions that protect the status quo. Plagiarism may persist because people with creative new ideas are continuously accepted into lower academic ranks, while those who plagiarize learn to cover their tracks with increasing skill and by using their influence.

Analyses of several studies and surveys have found that about 2% of scientists admit to plagiarism,

---

[503] Stark, L. & Perfect, T. (2007) Memory 15:776

[504] Hadid, A., op. cit; abusive attacks on a young author accompanied by plagiarism are a mark of authoritative status.

[505] See LaFollette, M. (1992) Stealing Into Print, for further discussion of plagiarism. Intelligent plagiarism persists strongly; occupants of academic hierarchies acquire novel ideas in many ways, such as asserting it was already stated by so-in-so, when in fact this is a bluff.

while 30% have observed plagiarism by their colleagues.[506] While this particular analysis shows that the rate of self-reported plagiarism has supposedly diminished, plagiarism observed in others has not, which may be the only honest observation of supposedly 'objective' self reports. Intelligent plagiarism modifies original material with contaminants that may be mistakes and have little long-term value, but are lost in the high quantity of publications of incremental and minor importance that are in journals. As broached here, can one fight plagiarism after the fact by publishing an improved theory with more explicit evidence to a discerning audience willing to read it, without attracting rephrased versions or offshoots of the theory by groups with more coauthors, resources and funding?

Official inquiries issued reports on the original 1986 paper basic to this book; as exercises in wordsmithing, these did not address the real issue of intellectual theft but discussed vague and diversionary considerations, which is to be expected if plagiarism is common and academic empathy is limited to colleagues of equal rank. Conformists ignore the persons who conceive diverse ideas but are prevented from participating in their implementation. Stereotypes are enforced by those with a bureaucratic attitude that confounds their status with rightful credit to the hidden sources of intellectual property. In my opinion, arguments distilled into coverups, allow offenders to continue to receive credit and funding for misappropriated intellectual property. This is another conflict of interest in academia, between allowing originators to slowly develop their own ideas, versus using large academic resources and expertise

---

[506] Pupovac, V. & Fanelli, D. (2014) Science Engin. Ethics; published online October 29.

to quickly bulldoze unknowns aside or to work around the explicit wording of patents, which is less expensive in time and money than brainstorming original, independent lines of thought.

There is a primeval biological need to allow those in power to maintain a stereotyped status, in front of a respectful public. However, this writer was in recent years in a room full of witnesses to a 'shaming' of a professor, apparently a result of years of secrecy at the highest academic levels. No public record of this verbal 'shaming' exists because universities and professors, in keeping with long experience, are adept at covering up to maintain a clean public image, as recent news reports suggest.[507] Additionally, labor rules can be used to penalize academics who accuse colleagues with specific evidence of misbehavior, so much so that a recent speaker who discussed these issues forbade any audio or video recording of the lecture. A disadvantage of the internet is that online documentation is modifiable at a later date, using any plausible excuse, to alter documentation giving evidence of use of specific ideas. In contrast to this non-transparent behavior, academics create a public relations impression of intellectual freedom to encourage diverse ideas that can enrich the environment of cohesive peers. Research on how groups acquire creative thinking from hidden individuals is phrased in bland language,[508] which shields plagiarism from official or public scrutiny.

---

[507] Fuller, T. (2016) New York Times March 24 and April 28, online edition. Reports are of coverups of sexual harassment and of conflicts of interest by a law school dean and a university chancellor.

[508] Nemeth, C., Personnaz, B., Personnaz, M., Goncalo, J. (2004) Eur. J. Social Psych. $\underline{34}$: 365; they show that social conflict, rather than a lack of criticism, results in creative solutions. Kim, S., Vincent, L., Goncalo, J. (2013) J. Exp. Psych. $\underline{142}$:605; this research measures how social independence increases creative expression.

This discussion is limited to anonymized generalities so that this book can be published without repression, though censorship can be easily disguised. Knockoffs of this theory by hidden readers may emerge that 'popularize' or rephrase it without referencing it, or reword original ideas without attribution. The time required to respond to transgressions by those with more resources, could be better spent producing and implementing logically consistent theories and new ideas, in future revisions.

Since I have found that plagiarism includes collusion between colleagues in different universities and departments, the focus should be on a structural cure for nuanced forms of plagiarism. For example, a paper, or its ideas, will be privately circulated without permission and used to design experiments, which the experimenter does not credit because this would reveal the deception. Or a friendly colleague may be leaked confidential information to develop and publish the ideas originated by another, which is then used as the reference. Sycophantic graduate students may also be fed the unpublicized idea to 'invent' in a thesis or initial publication. Vaguer versions of the ideas may be published that are not directly traceable to the originator.[509] The most damaging form of plagiarism for scientists lies outside of the scope of copyright protection; the insight or idea is retained but surrounded with different evidence, phrasing and/or new terminology.[510] I have found that recent transgressors subtly misappropriate

---

[509] Everyone 'in the know' is aware who originated a good idea, but this knowledge is not often publicized. Subtle hierarchical distinctions are important in academia; so if a work with important ideas is not published, it may not be credited unless the originator is a friend.

[510] Biagioli, M. (2012) Intl. J. Cultural Prop. 19:453; this author's recent publications also detail increasingly sophisticated forms of scientific plagiarism and fraud.

ideas by performing incrementally more cohesive experiments, which do not acknowledge that they are testing the 1986 idea of convergent neural spatial stability, even though they have tentatively communicated with the originator. The acquisition of a theory can also be disguised by copying the relevant facts initially, then sequentially adding the linking ideas that bind them, as if in a natural progression. In my opinion, this hidden use of insightful ideas or theories should be credited. Unilateral decisions by those in control disrespect the originator who then wants no association with such bold plagiarism. An overestimated self-importance in those who occupy hierarchical layers of authority[511] facilitates the plagiarism of persons with less status.

A primal competition for hierarchy dominates human evolution. The ever-evolving spiral of hacker efforts that attempt to supersede changing computer security procedures shows this incremental hand-over-hand cycling for dominance. Kurt Godel formalized this lack of a superseding metalogic as the Incompleteness Theorem. This circularly consistent logic is similar to the Anthropic Principle, in which the physical conditions that create life are embodied in the specific values of the physical constants of the universe, allowing the observer to perceive his own existence. The egocentric observer of Chapters Three and Four, has a perceptual moment that impedance matches, or synchronizes, with the standard physical constants measured externally.

The last paragraph should support induction, in which logical principles are made general, rather than a solipsistic view through rose-colored glasses. The mirroring of confirmatory logic, points to a sys-

---

[511] Duguid, M. & Goncalo, J. (2012) Psych. Sci. $\underline{23}$:36.

temic circular thinking basic to science, akin to the pre-selection by biased scientific techniques discussed earlier in this chapter. The Anthropic Principle is inductively consistent with one scientific standard, sensed by each egocentric observer or singular experimental apparatus. This circularity means no metalogic exists in applied science because existing scientists, due to their hierarchy, are arbitrarily designated as final authorities, who not only determine what is publishable, but some may rephrase it for their own credit. No checks and balances, division of powers or democratic process exists that could alter the consensus views of decision makers to create disincentives for hidden plagiarism.

To establish a neurophysiological theory, this chapter has stated that it is necessary to reassess the tried and true methodologies that have worked historically, to reexamine data so that it is driven to more creative solutions. The theory described here is more consistent with experimental results than the current information theory that interprets spikes as bits of data. We have become so adapted to fragmentary facts and incomplete lines of thought that it may be difficult to comprehend that logically consistent integrations exist. If visual system anatomy is fixed and identical spikes summate at repeated synaptic stages, and these phenomena are robust with a high confidence level, then this theory also has a high level of confidence.

While some parts of the theory do not have direct support, correctly designed experiments may fill the gaps where ambiguity now exists. For example, how does a precise, rapid reemission of spikes result in rapid IT cortical categorization of an object, but slower temporal summation of sustained input result in either a gist or more precise identification? How do spatially and temporally coincident z inputs on the same convergent V1/V2 cells, reemit synchronously as sequential motion or as a stable visual image? If neurophysiology evolves from statistical averages of data to more precisely described spike routes between synapses in individual neurons, the theory developed here may have more experimental support. Rather than top-down science standards that bias the interpretation of data, one must use basic biological data (which here is composed of identical spikes in labeled neural routes) to develop a theory with internal and experimental consistency.

The present top-down reductionist approach in science introduces bureaucratic layers in which status and authority confound with objectivity. A major research paradigm is parceled out to followers, who devise experiments based on increasingly specialized learning, with their smaller bit of the pie.[512] Historically retained templates increase the incremental complexity of new knowledge that still requires old knowledge as a foundation. Serially advanced degrees require incremental advances that conform with stabilized knowledge standards, which discourages the emergence of disruptive ideas.

An improved objectivity compares incremental experiments based on one interpretation, versus diverse interpretations of experiments with differing methods. But in an age of summaries, abstracts, synopses and metaanalyses of aggregated studies, subtleties of logic specific to experimental conditions may be ignored in favor of simplifications necessary to aggregate massive quantities of data. Parsing data may yield insights specific to time and place,

---

[512] Maher, B. & Sureda-Anfres, M. (2016) Nature 538:444; competition has increased for smaller rewards.

but data complexity increases costs in time, resources and interpretational complexity.

An easily accessible, well-publicized, non-hackable protocol now exists to rapidly publish original material on line, reducing the risk that confidential ideas are pirated from them by secret readers. The risk that unpublished material is secretly disseminated can now be replaced with open review of preprints online.[513] However, any online or other published material can be censored simply by an unwillingness to acknowledge unfamiliar concepts by influencers who follow standardized scripts, which keeps current research and grants from being outdated. Scientific material is now so complex, or in this book multidisciplinary, that it requires layers of specialized peer reviewers, further displacing the fragmentary experiment and its data from the observer. Aggregated layers increase the probability for distortions.

To decrease the importance of a scientific bureaucracy whose structure does not generate independent thinking, requires a more pluralistic approach, as espoused in a recent book.[514] Rapid internet communication increases the cohesion of groups that inhibit unconventional expression.[515] If a hierarchy akin to animal societies requires the top-down imposition of layered ranks to preserve the established scientific standards and self-interests of authority, it should also reduce incrementally introduced biases, such as excessive hype, officious plagiarism and fi-

---

[513] See websites biorxiv.org, arXiv.org and F1000Research.com.

[514] Excellent Sheep: The Miseducation of the American Elite (2014) by William Deresiewicz. This author decries the lack of thinking ability in the graduates of top universities.

[515] Lanier, J. (2006) Beware the Online Collective, in Edge.org. 'Democratic' rule must not be a majority that is an entitled mob.

nancial influence, which contaminate overall objectivity. Tactical increases in complexity and accrual of power to larger scientific entities that ignore ethical considerations, may reach a tipping point where a strategic change occurs that is not foreseen.

An objectivity based on unchanging standards should be realized as a tree with a robust trunk of evidence. For logic to be sequential, a complete neuroanatomical and physiological knowledge should be established at an appropriate level of complexity, before studies that depend on its stability are instituted. Otherwise interim theories and interpretations become outdated or more complex, as overlooked anatomical and physiological details are exposed. It may be asserted that innovation should be due to originality, not due to incrementally added data by new techniques that alter standards or add complexity. Previous discussion of Eyal et al. (op. cit. Chapter 4) has shown that experimental design and the degree of analysis or synthesis, profoundly affects the results obtained and their interpretation. Hidden metaphysical or operational assumptions have to be questioned so that they are also robust. Standardized 'Time' as a generic substrate to transmit temporally coded information, as discussed in this book, is one such assumption.

The increase in interpretational complexity of large data is exacerbated by scientists studying the same phenomenon with similar protocols but without the transparency and translatability necessary to replicate results.[516] Multiple understandings and interpretations of the same phenomenon result (see Motter & Poggio vs. Gur & Snodderley, in Chapter Three). Massive data, upon integration into sys-

---

[516] Capes-Davis, A., Neve, R. (2016) PLoS Biol. 14:e1002477.

tems biology simulations, creates irreproducible results, despite standardized procedures.[517] Perhaps complex simulations cannot replicate, in which slight differences in precision can magnify into large errors over many algorithmic iterations.

As stated, theoretical simplicity can perhaps accrue with interdisciplinary collaborations that integrate formerly fragmented efforts to resolve experimental and interpretational inconsistencies. Paradoxically, comprehensive theories like the one developed here, can resolve apparent anomalies by redefining at an appropriate level of hierarchical complexity. The idea here that identical spikes do not encode detailed image information is a simpler idea, yet one that may not be seen as 'scientific' by a discriminating science that analyzes a problem into smaller, solvable parts. Questions still exist that may have simpler solutions, despite the layers of increasingly complex, data-rich analyses that will continue to increment ad infinitum. This treatise has shown that the assumptions and perspectives of observers can determine a path with less inevitable complexity that creates insightful solution of the problem. Should we alter the research engine that is hierarchically driven to smaller bits of more complex knowledge, for more integrative research based on the brain's mechanisms, and so redefine epistemological boundaries?

---

[517] Waltemath, D., Wolkenhauer, O. (2016) IEEE Trans. Biomed. Engin. published before print online.

www.ingramcontent.com/pod-product-compliance
Lightning Source LLC
Chambersburg PA
CBHW050049230526
45470CB00004B/1458